The Pharmacy Guide To Herbal Remedies

The Pharmacy Guide to Herbal Remedies

Jan de Vries

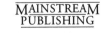

MAINSTREAM
PUBLISHING

EDINBURGH AND LONDON

First published in Great Britain in 2001 by
MAINSTREAM PUBLISHING COMPANY (EDINBURGH) LTD
7 Albany Street
Edinburgh EH1 3UG

Reprinted 2003

ISBN 1 84018 372 1

A catalogue record for this book is available
from the British Library

Typeset in Footlight and Garamond
Printed and bound in Great Britain by
Creative Print and Design Wales

THE PRODUCTS OF THE EARTH BEING OUR LIFE,
WHY NOT THE PRODUCTS OF THE EARTH OUR MEDICINE?

CONTENTS

INTRODUCTION

In front of me is a little book, written by an unknown author. There is no date to say when the book was written, though I think that it must have been at the end of the 1800s. What intrigued me about this book was the story of the Rt. Hon. W.E. Gladstone and botany, and the following extract from a speech he made at Guy's Hospital in London on 26 March 1890.

The origin of the medical profession was traceable to two sources – the first was the observation of nature which produced the herbalist . . . He was not aware whether botany now formed a recognised branch of medical education. He could not help wishing it did, because not only was it in itself a most beautiful and interesting study, exercising the mind without fatiguing it, and stimulating the imagination without leading it astray, but it led to a careful observation of nature, and to a habit of noticing the qualities of plants which were remarkable and so powerful in their healing capacity. Perhaps his hearers would think it almost ludicrous if he told a little anecdote of his own, which, simple and slight though it was, illustrated what he meant. As was pretty well known, he had been given to the pursuit of woodcutting. One day, by pure accident, he drew his finger along a tolerably large bit of the edge of his axe, and cut his finger. On searching about him he found he had no pocket handkerchief available. He wanted to staunch his little wound. He got a leaf and put it on. He was bound to say that it was not the result of botanical knowledge; it was strictly an empirical proceeding. But the curious result

> was the healing of this little breach of continuity
> occupied exactly half the time unassisted nature would
> have required. It was perhaps hardly worth
> mentioning, but he could not help thinking that there
> were great treasures in nature more than had
> heretofore been explored in that as in every other
> branch. – *Daily News*, 27 March 1890

Herbal medicine is as old as Creation, going back to the time when God promised man food to exist and herbs for healing, back to the time when there was no other medicine but herbal medicine. We still, however, have not discovered all that nature has to offer. We have spent billions discovering the Moon, and yet we have not researched all that is growing on Earth. There are herbs, plants, trees, woods and barks around the world that have never been researched and which I believe will have great healing powers.

In the Karolinska Institute in Stockholm, which houses the oldest medical library in the world, we find information on herbal remedies, many of which – like in the herbalist's anecdote – were discovered by accident, often without help or financial aid.

I was in a fortunate position when I bought the oldest herbal pharmacy in Edinburgh, Napiers, which had been owned by generations of botanists or pharmacists: in the old cellar I found remedies and recipes that had been used in the days of the plague. I use them on twentieth-century diseases, some of which are said to be incurable, and these remedies or combinations have given me great results. I was also fortunate when I bought an old herbalist practice in England, Abbotts of Leigh: there too I found books and prescriptions used in the 1800s which have given me many surprises in all that nature has to offer. Pharmacy has come a long way, and I never thought, when I graduated as a young pharmacist in 1958, that my way of life would follow the paths it has.

I still remember descending the stairs with my certificate closely clutched to my chest, being congratulated by the Minister of Health as the youngest graduate in pharmacy history. I had a head full of knowledge – or probably nonsense – of how I could relieve human suffering. But I also knew then that I could never take part in the explosion of antibiotics, tranquillisers and strong-acting drugs. I wondered if I could use my training to do something more with nature? This was probably ingrained in me, as I am descended from a long line of families which practised herbal medicine. When I became a practising pharmacist, I noticed that people came in simply to buy 100 capsules of garlic or to ask for a prescription of half chamomile, half sage – which is wonderful for colds and flu. Some would ask for a mixture of half liquid honey and half cod liver oil to cure an open leg ulcer. And these people came back because the remedies worked. I realised then, in 1958, how rapidly drugs were being developed and also how interested people were in herbal or natural remedies.

Pharmacies in Holland, where I come from, operate differently from those in Britain, where I now live. The pharmacist had the right to make up prescriptions, and the druggist was allowed to sell over-the-counter remedies. The pharmacists was highly qualified and well paid, often more than a doctor. Then the law on making up medications in pharmacies changed. Medications came pre-packed, and the druggist took over a large part of the pharmacist's business. This was a worrying development. I had often thought about how the development of natural remedies could benefit patients and I started to introduce some herbal and homoeopathic remedies. I started in a small way because I was still a bit sceptical; nevertheless I could not argue with the results. Gradually I introduced many of my grandmother's remedies. And now that I have been almost forty years in practice, I know why complementary medicine is growing so fast.

Not long ago I was asked to write an article for the UK weekly *Chemist & Druggist.* Before I wrote that article I did some research and what I found gave me a shock. One big pharmacy that I visited had devoted most of its shelf space to goods with brand names like Houbigant, Guerlain, Elizabeth Arden, Lancôme and Christian Dior; indeed, much of its business came from selling fragrances and cosmetics. I went to another, smaller pharmacy and found it richly stocked with washing powders and sanitary products. These pharmacies had very small dispensaries manned by the pharmacist. A pharmacist knows his responsibilities; he also has a solid education behind him, and I said to myself, 'Is this what pharmacy is all about?'

The pharmacist can play an important role advising patients. Doctors are often very busy, and the patient is often scared to ask for information, so the pharmacist is the next person for the patient to run to for help. The question is: is he available? Has he time? Is he interested in giving the information that is necessary? This is a big gap in the British market. The gap has been partially filled by the health food stores; indeed, a lot of people go to the trained health food shop managers with their questions. But the health food shops (called reform shops in Holland) are restricted in the products that they are allowed to sell. In Holland (and also in Germany, Switzerland and France) when the laws on making up medication in pharmacies changed, many pharmacists saw their turnover dwindle and diversified. Some set up information centres, some, like myself, studied complementary medicine in order to advise their patients and customers, and others started their own pharmacies with treatment rooms or information centres.

I was aware of the huge market potential when I did the postgraduate course for pharmacists in Northern Ireland. My heart soared when I went to the offices of the National Pharmaceutical Society and saw showcases containing herbs and concoctions, ointments and salves that we used to make in pharmacy. Why are the old herbal remedies coming back? The millennium pharmacist knows that they are part of the range of medications available and is aware that, by using his knowledge, he can increase his ability to advise the public. The public knows that pharmacists are under oath to do what is right and that the remedies which the pharmacist advises will have few or no side effects. In this book I have written about remedies that I have used for forty years in my ten successful practices, and the knowledge that I have gathered from all over the world.

It was a most fortunate occasion when, in 1959, I attended a lecture on homoeopathy given by Professor Zabal in Amsterdam. Next to me was a gentleman who, during the break, asked me what I thought of homoeopathy. 'Well, it is all right for old spinsters and vegetarians,' I replied. He then said something that stuck in my mind: 'You must have a very small mind.' The gentleman was right. I knew very little about the subject, and his retort made me interested in what he had to say.

This gentleman was Dr Alfred Vogel, who was a guru of alternative medicine in those days. He told me of the benefits that people would find from herbal remedies. He invited me to his home in Switzerland and took me to the clinics of Bircher Benner, Issel's clinic and other places. To my great joy he took me up into the mountains, sometimes 6,000 feet high, to teach me all about herbs and plants and their benefits. Even better, we went out with a group of gypsies who shared much of their knowledge about what was growing there. They became my best teachers. These times often reminded me of a period during the

Second World War when my mother was heavily involved in the Dutch resistance and we were in Arnheim, Oosterbeek. Every day she would send me next door to an old monastery, where the old monk in charge of the herbal garden taught me much about plants and which herbs were used to help people.

These experiences made me want to study again. I started studying complementary medicine (and I continued studying until I was 54). I learned and learned. When Dr Vogel and I started the first clinic of nature cure at the beginning of the 1960s, I was really involved with the patients. Today, pharmacy plays a big role in relieving human suffering. I am happy that pharmacists now see the need for natural medicine.

Some years ago, when I worked with Boots on a project, I said then that natural remedies would become the preferred choice of many people. And certainly on the many radio and television programmes that I have done, I have had positive feedback from thousands of people. I feel, therefore, that I have a duty to pass on my knowledge and experiences; hence, this is my thirtieth book. This is the first of a series of books on subjects that are of particular interest to pharmacy today. It has two main parts. The first part, 'Regularly Prescribed Herbal Products', lists some of the branded products that I have used most often in my practices. It describes their properties and explains when and how to use them. The second part, 'Herbal and Homoeopathic Remedies', suggests herbal and homoeopathic remedies that might be useful for particular medical conditions or to help to restore and heal the body. The final sections contain useful information: summaries of clinical trials of three herbal remedies, safety advice for people using St John's wort and a glossary of medical terms.

There are thousands of preparations that I could have chosen for treating various ailments, but I have confined my selection to those that I have seen working effectively and without any side effects. Some of them are single herbal remedies, others are combinations. Thankfully we don't have to mix our own preparations as in the old days. For instance, for a headache, you had to boil 1oz scullcap, 1oz rosemary, 1oz taraxacum herb, 1oz menthe viride and 1oz verbena herb in a quart of water for three minutes, strain the liquid and, when cold, drink a wineglassful three times a day. Or to keep the bowels regular, make pills from 2 drachms solid extract cascara, 2 drachms lobelia herb, 2 drachms turkey rhubarb, 2 drachms extract of dock and take one or two of these pills before bedtime three nights a week, and indulge in as much fresh air as possible. It is a lot easier now that there are pre-packed herbal remedies that serve the same purpose.

In this book I have endeavoured to give enough guidance for pharmacists to feel safe and confident to give advice to customers on the remedy needed to resolve whatever problems they may have. However, as I have stressed so often before, guidance is necessary and it is always important for patients to consult a GP, herbalist or qualified practitioner for the necessary assistance.

There are, of course, several ways in which we can look at remedies, and at least two different ways in which a remedy can work. My great friend Dr Hans Mollenburg, from Haarlem, Holland, once gave a lecture on the two ways in which remedies can work. He said that:

1. We can look at it the pharmacological way. This is the usual way we are taught at university. A tranquilliser alters something in your brain in a chemical way and can make you as tame as a toy dog. Antidepressants, antibiotics, antihypertensive drugs all work in a chemical way. They change something inside your body. They are Active and you are Passive.

2. The information way. These remedies are no more or less than a message. They are like a telephone call to police HQ to say that there might be a burglary taking place in Baker Street. It calls out the police force, but in itself it has no power. I am not talking about a placebo effect here. Active immunisation acts this way, as do homoeopathic remedies, Bach remedies or other flower remedies. When you give the whole plant, as we usually do in a herbal treatment, the same principle is at work. There is, of course, also a plain pharmacological activity, but the information part in my view is quite strong. The plant gives the body a message, telling it how to cope with a certain problem. They activate the body's own resistance.

So in my view, herbal remedies are a mixture of 1 and 2.

What sort of message do they give? In the laboratory of Dr Hauschka, scientists took extracts of three different species of roses and dropped each of the rose extracts onto the middle of a piece of finely grained filter paper, which had been impregnated with metal salts. The rose extracts formed stylised flowers on the back of the filter paper; however, each of the species of rose had its own specific structure on the paper. This experiment is repeatable. However, plants lose this structuring capacity when they have been artificially fertilised or sprayed with insecticides. So you could say that a message is there: the message of the structure. But there is more. When a copper chloride solution crystallises, the crystals lie in a zigzag formation on the plate. When you add a herbal extract to the solution, the structure is fundamentally altered. And when you add a solution from leaves that are already dead the structure begins to deteriorate. A slide of sick nerve tissue would look chaotic in structure. If you added monkshood plant, which has a strong regenerative action on nerve tissue, the monkshood would remind the body of the correct structure; it would pull the nerve back to normal.

Bach Flower Remedies consist mainly of these messages on a mental level. Once there was a patient who nearly suffocated on his way into my consulting room. I asked if something had happened and he said, 'I am full of hate. I hate my ex-wife who keeps my daughter away from me. I want to kill her.' I gave this man holly, for those who hate. Ten days later his condition had improved. I asked him about his hate and he said, 'You know, in my head I know I should hate her but I do not feel it anymore.' So what could be the message of holly? Not love, love is not the opposite of hate. The opposite of love is indifference. Could it be eternity, perhaps? Seeing suddenly that puny hate is rather unimportant in the vastness of our universe. In my opinion, when we work with herbal remedies we should not only have the pharmacological knowledge, but also this other way of looking at them, trying to find their message.

When working with herbal remedies we should realise that we work with living entities. An iscador (or mistletoe extract) injection gives a different feeling to that of a chemotherapy injection. The stories surrounding mistletoe give this plant flesh and blood and coming across it in nature is like meeting an old friend. When you feel like that towards a herbal remedy it works better. In the case of iscador it does far more than just inhibiting the growth of a tumour. It is a fact that people who receive this treatment often open up. They begin to produce important dreams, they begin to cry, and they begin to talk about life and death. Iscador is not only a tumour inhibitor; it is also a plant giving an important message. The message is live!

I have emphasised how unscientific herbal therapy really is. Making herbal tea is far more like composing a piece of music than using medical technology. It is connected with ancient knowledge: the art of healing. Let's look at St John's wort. When you look at the leaves against the light they appear to have holes punched around them. That is why the plant is called *Hypericum perforatum*. The 'holes' are in fact tiny oil glands and the oil, although you cannot see it when it is still in the leaf, is a blood-red colour. Does St John's wort work? Yes, it does. It is a natural tranquilliser. We all know that it is not easy to reprogramme the mind. We must first make it rest, and often this cannot be done by mental exercises; the mind is too much like a monkey swinging from branch to branch. Often we go round and round vicious circles. 'Is this pain cancer? I daren't go to the doctor. He might find a cancer. I will have to go to the hospital. Perhaps I will die in pain. I will not go to the doctor. But I definitely feel pain. Is this pain cancer?' Sometimes patients involve me in their vicious circles, like one lady who came to see me.

'With your gallbladder problem you must stop eating chocolate, madam.'

'But I like chocolate so much.'

'Yes, but it may give you another attack, you'd better not eat it.'

'But I simply cannot resist chocolate. I must have it.'

'Then by all means eat it.'

'How can you tell me to eat chocolate, doctor, when you know perfectly well it is bad for me?'

How does St John's wort work? It chases away thoughts that could be harmful to you. The message of St John's wort is: relax, let go, be at ease. Could one say that in the signature of this plant there is an indication that it works the way we know it does? Take the most striking characteristic of this plant. Hold the leaf against the light. It is as if minuscule pieces of light have been trapped in the leaf. It should be a light spender. So if one wants to enlighten a situation, be it to relax a muscle or to enlighten a burdened mind, remember St John's wort.

I know there has been a lot of criticism of St John's wort. Often when a product becomes very popular it comes under attack. In forty years of practice, however, I have never seen any side effects when taken in its fresh extract form. It is sensible when taking long-term medication such as warfarin or aspirin to take advice from a GP. You cannot use herbal remedies in the same way as you would remedies from a chemical factory. There is an extra dimension in herbal therapy and if you do not realise it, you miss a lot. This might conflict with your training. In this day and age a remedy is recognised only when we can find the active substances with a clear pharmacological action. We have, for instance, extracted the active ingredient in foxglove. Our happiness is complete when we can synthesise the compound. And, yes, the action on the heart is there with the synthetic product, but what happened to the message? In some plants the active ingredient has not been isolated and thus they are discarded. But you can safely bet that when a herbal remedy has been in use for a couple of thousand years it is a healing plant, even if the healing factor is unknown. The probability is that its action is mainly message-like and not pharmacological.

In the first chapter of this book I shall describe some of the herbal remedies I have worked with for many years. When I was with Dr Vogel in the Alps I learned about these remedies and many times saw their characteristics. I remember standing on some arnica. Dr Vogel stopped me. 'Did you hear it?' he asked. 'It talked back to you.' Arnica makes a noise when you step on it, as if to say, 'Please, watch out!' I take arnica when there is trauma or bruising. I remember a conversation with the Queen in which she told me that her grandfather always carried arnica in his pocket in case anything happened. He would use it for immediate help. Look at echinacea, which Dr Vogel did so much to promote when he discovered the terrific immunity of the plant. I remember an old man in North America telling me to put a bunch of echinacea in a vase and they would flower for a long time, even without water. They have immunity and today are recognised as one of the finest and strongest antibiotics. While in North America, we saw some hamamelis branches growing. The native Americans brought the medicinal virtues of *Hamamelis virginiana*, or witch hazel, to the notice of European settlers. It was included in the US *Pharmacopoeia* in 1882. Hamamelis is from the Greek *hama*, together, and *melon*, an apple, as flowers and fruit are produced at the same time. The plant has many wonderful constituents, which can be used as an astringent and haemostatic. It is useful for nosebleeds, insect bites, sweaty feet as well as diarrhoea and dysentery.

And so one can go on. Let us now look at the benefits and uses of some of the remedies that I have prescribed for so many years.

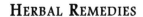
This chapter is concerned with the herbal products that I have used most often – and successfully – in my practices. They cover a range of complementary therapies, including herbal medicine (phytotherapy), flower remedies and homoeopathy and are grouped by manufacturer. Each product is listed with information such as ingredients and usage. In deference to my former partner Dr Vogel, I shall start this chapter with the remedies that he developed and ones that I later helped with. But before I do, I shall say a little about phytotherapy.

The word 'phytotherapy' comes from the Greek *phyton*, meaning 'plant' or 'herb', and was used for the first time by the French physician Henri Leclerc (1879–1955). The therapy developed from centuries-old, traditional herbal medicine. However, progress from old herbal medicine to modern phytotherapy was slow: it took a long time – far too long – for the old herbal medicine to free itself of its many superstitions and use of herbal magic, which was so deeply rooted in the traditional healing practices of folk medicine.

Phytotherapy is the therapeutic application of healing and medicinal plants which are used in the preparation of remedies made of whole plants or parts thereof. It encompasses all plants, from the 'harmless' healing plants such as chamomile to the strongly effective such as digitalis or belladonna. The designation 'harmless' does not necessarily mean that these healing herbs are less effective. It means that these herbs produce no immediate or intensive effects and also that they do not possess a substantial toxicity, so that they may be administered over an extended period of time for therapeutic purposes without causing any harm.

Phytotherapy is not, however, homoeopathy; the application of herbal medicines according to homoeopathic principles is fundamentally different from phytotherapy. Nevertheless, phytotherapy owes much of its inspiration to homoeopathy, since a great number of plants used in homoeopathy would otherwise hardly be known to herbal medicine.

Phytotherapy has established three basic rules, which have mainly grown out of practical experience:

1. **Application of 'harmless' healing herbs**
   It has been learned that much can be achieved with simple, therapeutic remedies, provided one has control over the technique of application and is able to properly prescribe the method of such application.
2. **Application of whole plant**
   Scientific research has always aimed to isolate the essential substances of a healing plant. The practical conclusion that was drawn, namely, to use only these essential substances, in practice has proven to be far less correct than one might have assumed. With most healing plants it is not just one individual principal substance that is effective but the totality of effective substances; that is, all the ingredients of the plant. Beyond these, there are a large number of healing plants that contain no principal essential substance at all but the totality of all the ingredients actually produce a therapeutic effect.
3. **Long-term, therapeutic application of healing plants**
   This rule applies to those plants whose effectiveness does not lie in strongly potent substances and which, therefore, do not display considerable immediate effectiveness. The healing effect takes place slowly after regular application over an extended period of time.

Phytotherapy has taken a huge step forward in the past decade. Two facts are especially significant in this regard. Firstly, scientific research has concerned itself increasingly with the use of herbs therapeutically and has achieved some remarkable results. Secondly, phytotherapy has developed more and more into a science in its own right. Many new developments have earned phytotherapy a new, improved reputation. In contrast to chemical, synthetic drugs, herbal medicines have remained close to nature or, if you will, close to people.

BIOFORCE

Alfred Vogel (1902–96) was a renowned nutritionist, herbalist, naturopath and author of many books and articles. The paramount figure in natural medicine, he devoted his life to the philosophy of living 'In Harmony with Nature'. He firmly believed that everything we needed to protect and preserve our health has been given to us by nature.

During his childhood, Vogel learnt about the therapeutic value of plants from his parents. In 1933 he established a naturopathic practice in the beautiful Swiss mountain village of Teufen, where he cultivated his own medicinal herbs.

Through his work, Vogel found that herbal preparations made from fresh plant materials were more beneficial to his patients than those medicines prepared using dried herbs. At Teufen he developed his theory further, producing herbal tinctures from fresh plants cultivated in the herb garden or collected from the surrounding mountains.

In 1963 he founded Bioforce, which manufactures the following remedies.

❦ AESCULUS ❦

Description
A herbal extract made from the fresh seeds of *Aesculus hippocastanum* (horse chestnut tree).

Aesculus has been used for venous conditions since the end of the nineteenth century. It is a tall tree with large sticky buds and seed that are instantly recognisable to many children who spend their autumn afternoons seeking out the biggest and best 'conkers' to thread onto a piece of string.

The origin of the generic name *Aesculus* is unclear. The species name, *hippocastanum*, literally means 'horse chestnut'. This term probably arose from the early use of the seed to treat coughing and broken wind in horses, distinguishing it from the chestnuts eaten by humans.

The use of Aesculus in venous disorders has been recognised for a long time. In the past, Aesculus was also used as an ingredient in snuff to treat nasal polyps. Prior to this, many people believed that carrying horse chestnut seeds in one's pocket would prevent gout, rheumatism and back pains.

Mode of action
Anti-inflammatory; astringent (tones blood vessels); anti-oedema.

Several constituents of Aesculus are important therapeutically; these include saponins (aescin), flavonoids, tannins and coumarins. The clinical action of Aesculus in peripheral venous disorders appears to depend on a number of these constituents rather than just one.

Flavonoids exhibit an anti-inflammatory action. Tannins have astringent properties, helping to tone the vessel walls.

Aescin is the constituent that appears to have the ability to inhibit oedema. It possesses anti-inflammatory action and increases venous tone. In varicose veins, aescin can influence the initial phase of inflammation by exerting a 'sealing' effect on 'leaky' capillaries, reducing both the number and diameter of capillary pores. It also inhibits the activity of lysosomal enzymes, which have the ability to damage the walls of veins and capillaries.

Dosage information
ADULTS: 20 drops in a little water twice a day immediately after meals. For maintenance, 20 drops in a little water once a day.
CHILDREN: It is unlikely that this product would be indicated for children.

> Aesculus should be taken immediately after meals. This reduces the possibility of gastrointestinal irritation by the saponin content.

Duration of administration
Longer-term use is advisable for best results.

Restrictions on use
None known.

Contra-indications
None known.

Pregnancy and nursing
No restrictions known. However, those who are pregnant or breastfeeding should consult a practitioner before using Aesculus.

Adverse reactions
Due to its coumarin content, Aesculus may interfere with anticoagulant therapy (for example, warfarin).

Ingredients
Aesculus hippocastanum 100 per cent
(Alcohol content: approximately 58 per cent)

Application
Venous tonic; varicose veins (varicose eczema, varicose ulcers); haemorrhoids; thread veins; phlebitis (inflammation of veins).

Disturbances in the venous circulation occur mainly in the lower extremities due to the greater pressure exerted on these veins.

Varicose veins and haemorrhoids appear when veins lose their elasticity. Blood then accumulates, causing distension and swelling of these blood vessels. Fluid is then forced into the surrounding tissue, giving rise to oedema. This can impede the circulation further, reducing tissue nutrition. In the legs, if this process is prolonged, varicose eczema results. This area of devitalised tissue becomes prone to damage. If trauma does occur, the healing process is protracted, giving rise to varicose ulcers.

Varicose veins and haemorrhoids are prone to inflammation (phlebitis). Many cases of night cramps arise as a result of poor venous circulation.

🦋 AGNUS CASTUS 🦋

Description
A tincture prepared from the fruit of *Agnus castus* (chaste tree), also known as *Vitex agnus-castus*.

Despite its common name, the chaste tree is actually a shrub. It has finger-like leaves, violet flowers and fruit which give off a pleasant peppermint-like smell due to volatile oils present.

In the past, *Agnus castus* has been used for rheumatic conditions and the common cold. However, it is now recognised that the strength of this herb in modern-day phytotherapy lies in its ability to influence the female reproductive hormones.

Mode of action
Acts at the level of the pituitary gland; increases the level of progesterone relative to oestrogen; inhibits prolactin.

Agnus castus acts on the pituitary gland to increase the secretion of lutenising hormone, which leads to the greater production of progesterone during the second half of the menstrual cycle.

This hormonal shift favouring progesterone helps to reduce premenstrual symptoms and alleviates menstrual disorders such as heavy menstrual bleeding and painful periods, which are related to higher oestrogen dominance.

Agnus castus has also been reported to have the ability to inhibit the action of prolactin. This is relevant in premenstrual syndrome as it has been postulated that many who suffer with this condition have a greater sensitivity to the hormone.

It has been suggested by some researchers that the prolactin inhibitory action of *Agnus castus* may be of help in the treatment of Parkinson's disease – a condition caused by a reduction in the amount of dopamine secreted by the substantia nigra, which then gives rise to difficulties with co-ordination and control of skeletal muscles. The metabolism of dopamine is intricately dependent on the amount of prolactin present. Reducing levels of prolactin reduces the rate of breakdown of dopamine in the brain, hence increasing the levels circulating in the tissue.

Agnus castus has been found to be beneficial in the treatment of acne in both men and women.

Dosage information
ADULTS: 15–20 drops in a little water twice a day.
ADOLESCENTS: 10–15 drops twice a day.

Duration of administration
Agnus castus is suitable for short- or long-term use.

Restrictions on use
Those using oral contraceptives or hormone replacement therapy (HRT) should ideally seek medical advice before using *Agnus castus.*

Contra-indications
We can find no contra-indications to the use of *Agnus castus* even in the early stages of puberty.

Pregnancy and nursing
It should not be taken during pregnancy unless under medical supervision.

Adverse reactions
Occasional skin rashes have been reported.

Ingredients
Agnus castus 100 per cent
(Alcohol content: approximately 69 per cent)

Application
Premenstrual syndrome; menstrual disorders (painful periods, heavy bleeding); acne; fibroids; endometriosis.

The premenstrual syndrome (PMS) is a condition which occurs between seven and 14 days before menstruation. It is characterised by a number of symptoms, which include decreased energy, tension, irritability, depression, headache, breast pain, backache, abdominal bloating and fluid retention.

PMS affects approximately one-third of women between the ages of 30 and 40. The underlying cause is thought to be an imbalance between oestrogen and progesterone in the menstrual cycle. It has also been suggested that high levels of prolactin, or an increased sensitivity to prolactin, may be implicated.

Agnus castus exerts a balancing effect on the activity of the female sex hormones. This activity may also be of benefit to those suffering fibroids and endometriosis.

❦ AVENA SATIVA ❦

Description
A traditional herbal 'nerve tonic' made from fresh oat seeds. It is known to have a nutritive and restorative action on the nervous system. It also has mild sedative and hypnotic properties.

Mode of action
Mild sedative; antidepressant.

Fresh oat seeds contain high amounts of vitamin B, minerals and other nutrients necessary for the proper functioning of the nervous system. These constituents probably account for the 'restorative' benefits in depression, states of debility and exhaustion.

Oats also contain indole alkaloids, the most active of which is gramine. These alkaloids have been shown to relax smooth muscles and exert a sedative action on the nervous system. It is of benefit to those suffering from chronic anxiety, hyperactivity and insomnia.

Research carried out by two Edinburgh doctors using the electroencephalograph (EEG) to assess sleep quality has shown that those using *Avena sativa* had a quieter sleep than those in the control group.

Oats is a safe remedy to use in children and its calming action can be of benefit in irritable and fractious children.

Despite being such a commonly used food, oats have a significant degree of sedative action. Anand found Ayurvedic physicians using oats to help with opium withdrawal. This led him to use the herb to aid nicotine withdrawal and he obtained good results treating 26 people heavily addicted to cigarettes. Others have used *Avena sativa* to help with the symptoms of withdrawal from alcohol and narcotic drugs.

Dosage information
ADULTS: 20 drops in a little water two or three times a day before meals.
CHILDREN: Half adult dose.
INFANTS: Two to five drops, two or three times a day.

Duration of administration
No restrictions on long-term usage known.

Restrictions on use
None known.

Contra-indications
None known.

Pregnancy and nursing
No restrictions known.

Adverse reactions
None known.

Ingredients
Avena sativa 100 per cent
(Alcohol content: approximately 43 per cent)
Other preparations in the Bioforce range containing *Avena sativa*: Ginsavena; Tormentil Complex.

Application
Nervous and mental exhaustion; depression/anxiety; teething infants; hyperactivity; reduces cravings.

The nervous system controls and integrates all the activities of the body – not only on a physical level but also on the psychological plane. The system may become debilitated and fatigued through factors such as stress, shock and faulty nutrition. In these circumstances a nerve tonic plays a useful role, strengthening, feeding and revitalising the system.

As *Avena sativa* is such a mild sedative, it may be used to calm young, fractious infants, particularly those distressed by colic or teething pains. It has been used successfully for the clinical treatment of hyperactivity in children, in conjunction with an appropriate diet.

Avena sativa has also been used to treat addiction – the most common form in our modern society is the dependence on nicotine. Withdrawal from this, or any other drug, would draw on both the psychological and physical reserves of the individual.

❦ BILBERRY ❦

Description
A fresh herbal extract of bilberry or European blueberry (*Vaccinium myrtillus*), which has been found to be of benefit in a number of conditions, but especially in maintaining health of the eyes.

Bilberry is a shrub that grows in woods and forests throughout Europe. The fruit is blue-black or purple and has a high nutritional value.

RAF pilots are said to have used bilberry (as well as carrots) to improve night-time vision for bombing raids.

Mode of action
Stimulates production of retinal pigments; collagen stabilising action; reduces capillary permeability; antioxidant; reduces blood glucose levels.

The main active constituents of bilberries appear to be flavoured compounds known as anthocyanosides. Each of these molecules consists of a 'core' molecule called anthocyanidin, which is bound to one of three sugars. Five different anthocyanidins may be found in bilberry, from which are derived more than 15 anthocyanosides.

A group of these anthocyanosides possess the ability to bind to the portion of the retina that is responsible for vision. This increases the rate of regeneration of the visual pigments in the retina, increasing the speed of adaptation to darkness.

Collagen is a protein which forms an important part of the body's corrective tissue. It provides tensile strength and integrity to the tissues of the body and, particularly, the eyes. The anthocyanidins in bilberry prevent the destruction of collagen, stabilising the tissue structures. This action is said to be important in the prevention and treatment of glaucoma.

Bilberry also contains bioflavonoids, which have the ability to increase vitamin C levels within cells. This in turn decreases capillary permeability and fragility, reducing the tendency for tissue damage and haemorrhage which may accompany many arterial, venous and capillary disorders such as diabetic retinopathy.

The anthocyanidin myrtillin has the additional action of reducing blood sugar levels. When administered by injection, this compound is said to possess action similar to that of insulin.

Dosage information
ADULTS: 20 drops in a little water twice a day before meals.
CHILDREN: It is unlikely that this product will be indicated for children.

Duration of administration
No restrictions on long-term use.

Restrictions on use
None known.

Contra-indications
None known.

Pregnancy and nursing
It is not recommended during pregnancy.

Adverse reactions
None known.

Ingredients
Vaccinium myrtillus 100 per cent
(Alcohol content: approximately 69 per cent)

Application
Eye strain (VDU operators); improves vision; protects against eye disorders; lowers blood sugar.

Good nutrition is important in maintaining the health of the eyes. A shortage of vitamin A may lead to poor vision, as this vitamin is essential in the formation of the retinal pigments responsible for vision. It has a protective effect on the eye surfaces and retina (by virtue of its antioxidant activity), tissues which are susceptible to damage by free radicals, produced through normal metabolic processes and sunlight.

Bilberry contains the antioxidant vitamins A and C, known to reduce the risk of cataracts. One study reported that the progression of cataract formation was halted in 97 per cent of patients treated with a mixture of bilberry and vitamin E.

The flavonoids present in the herb have been shown to improve the function of the retina, improving night vision and halting diabetic eye disease. In addition, this group of compounds has also been shown to possess hypoglycaemic action.

♥ CENTAURIUM ♥

Description
A herbal extract made from *Centaurium umbellatum* (centaury), which has been used as a stomach bitter for many years.

Centaurium is one of the most important stomach bitters available to us. It is part of the gentian family, Gentianaceae. Two other members of this family, *Gentiana lutea* (great gentian) and *Gentiana purpurea* (yellow gentian), also possess useful bitter properties.

Centaurium is a small, inconspicuous plant which grows in large numbers in dry grassy areas. It is a spiky plant with a small head of pink flowers. The herb is bitter to taste even when diluted in water to a ratio of 1:3,500.

In some countries the bitter properties of centaury are used in alcoholic and non-alcoholic beverages. It is listed by the Council of Europe as a natural food flavouring.

Mode of action
Bitter tonic; digestive stimulant.

Centaurium owes its action to the group of compounds called bitter glycosides. The taste of these substances in the mouth stimulates the appetite and triggers the secretion of digestive juices in the stomach. This in turn improves the breakdown of food.

At the same time, the hormone gastrin is secreted by the walls of the stomach. This enhances gastric motility and relaxes the pyloric sphincter, which allows food to pass out of the stomach more easily. At the same time, the tone of the oesophageal sphincter is increased, preventing reflux of food from the stomach back into the oesophagus, a process which is responsible for the symptoms of heartburn.

Centaurium also tones up a 'sluggish' digestion. It enhances the appetite – an action which may be beneficial in children who are 'picky eaters', adults recovering from illnesses, poor eaters or those suffering from anorexia nervosa.

Dosage information
ADULTS: Ten drops in a little water three times a day before meals.
CHILDREN: Half adult amount.

> An adjustment to the recommended dosages may be required due to individual differences in the sensitivity to bitter herbs. Ideally, Centaurium, like all bitter herbs, should be taken 15 minutes before meals. It should always be taken in a little water, sipped and held in the mouth before swallowing to stimulate its action.

Duration of administration
No restriction on long-term usage known.

Restrictions on use
None known.

Pregnancy and nursing
No restrictions known.

Adverse reactions
None known.

Ingredients
Centaurium umbellatum 100 per cent
(Alcohol content: approximately 63 per cent)

Application

General indigestion; gastric reflux (heartburn, hiatus hernia); anorexia (lack of appetite).

Stomach bitters are used to improve digestion. They do so by increasing the secretion of digestive enzymes and increasing gut motility. These actions, mediated via the hormone gastrin, enhance the breakdown of food which then helps to relieve symptoms of indigestion such as nausea, flatulence, fullness and gastric discomfort.

Another important function of gastrin is to tighten the oesophageal sphincter. This reduces the tendency for reflux of the gastric contents into the oesophagus, a condition which is seen with hiatus hernia and other causes of reflux which give rise to the symptom of heartburn.

The ability of Centaurium to improve the appetite in those with anorexia can be of use in both children and adults. It is worth while to note that this herb will not influence a normal appetite.

❧ CRATAEGUS ❧

Description

This preparation is made from the fresh fruits (berries) of hawthorn (*Crataegus oxyacantha*).

The hawthorn is a small spiny tree or shrub native to Europe. It can sometimes reach a height of 30 feet but it is often grown as a hedge plant. Hawthorn flowers and berries have been used for many years by phytotherapists as a 'heart tonic', being indicated for many conditions involving the heart and arterial circulation.

Mode of action

Improves coronary circulation (circulation to the heart); improves efficiency of heart muscle; calms the heart.

Crataegus has become one of the most widely used herbal remedies for the heart. Its precise mode of action is still being investigated, but one thing which has been established is that the herb is not a digitaloid – it does not contain digitalis-like compounds.

The main groups of active constituents in Crataegus have now been identified. Clinically, the action of the plant results from the balanced effect of all these constituents. However, a number of compounds have been found to play significant roles.

The flavonoids are primarily responsible for the vasodilatory effect on the coronary circulation, increasing blood flow to this vital organ. To a lesser extent, vasodilation also occurs in the peripheral circulation. The sum of these actions is a reduction in blood pressure, an improvement in the coronary circulation and a reduction in the likelihood of angina attacks.

Glycosides increase the tone of the heart, improving the force of contraction whilst reducing the rate of contraction. This improvement in functional efficiency makes Crataegus a useful heart tonic.

Dosage information
ADULTS: 15–20 drops in a little water three times a day.
CHILDREN: It is unlikely that this product will be indicated for
   children.

Duration of administration
Crataegus should be used for several months to benefit from its full effect. It is completely safe for long-term treatment. It is important not to discontinue a medically prescribed cardiovascular medication while taking it.

Restrictions on use
None known.

Contra-indications
None known.

Pregnancy and nursing
Not recommended without medical advice.

Interactions
It may be taken alongside pharmaceutical medicines, but may increase the action of preparations such as digoxin. For this reason, it is best to seek the advice of a doctor if Crataegus is to be used with existing 'heart medicines'.

Adverse reactions
None known.

Ingredients
Crataegus oxyacantha 100 per cent
(Alcohol content: approximately 43 per cent)

Other preparations containing Crataegus in the Bioforce range: Hawthorn–Garlic Complex.

Application
Heart tonic; angina; benign palpitations; arteriosclerosis (intermittent claudication); mild hypertension.

Crataegus has been used for many years as a 'heart tonic', being able to improve the efficiency of the pumping action of the heart. It does so by increasing blood flow in the coronary arteries (arteries supplying the muscles of the heart). These actions are important in many of the modern-day ailments affecting the heart.

The cardiovascular system is the term given to the heart, the arteries, veins and capillaries which are the conduits through which blood is transported throughout the body. When this system is working efficiently a constant circulation is maintained.

Many conditions may arise which can impede this flow. The commonest disorder of blood vessels is arteriosclerosis or hardening of the arteries, which can give rise to high blood pressure, angina and intermittent claudication.

❧ ECHINAFORCE ❧

Description
This preparation, made from the aerial parts and roots of *Echinacea purpurea*, is considered to be the prime herbal remedy for the immune system. This view has been supported by extensive research, confirming the traditional uses which were first recognised by native Americans.

Mode of action
Immune stimulant; anti-inflammatory; antiseptic; antiviral; antibacterial.

Echinacea is an immune stimulant. As a result of this, it has anti-inflammatory, antiviral and antibacterial activity associated with the polysaccharide and polyacetylene components present in the plant.

These constituents mobilise our defence mechanism by activating and stimulating the release of leucocytes (white blood cells), which fight infection. The function of T-lymphocytes is enhanced and there is an increase in the number of macrophages (which have phagocytic ability – the mechanism in which foreign material is engulfed and destroyed).

Echinacin, a polysaccharide, promotes wound healing by inhibiting the enzyme hyaluronidase. This helps to promote the growth of new tissue, activating fibroblasts which are the cells responsible for encouraging wound healing.

Three varieties of echinacea have been used by phytotherapists. Bauer, the German phytotherapy researcher, found that these species have differing activities. Using experimental methods which measured immune stimulation, he found that alcoholic extracts of *Echinacea purpurea* gave the greatest activity, followed by alcoholic extracts of *E. angustifolia* and *E. pallida*, which were 65 per cent less active.

Dosage information

ADULTS: 15 drops in a little water two or three times a day.

CHILDREN (6–12 years): Seven drops in a little water two or three times a day.

Extracts of *Echinacea purpurea* are available in tablet form and as a cream.

Duration of administration

If Echinaforce is needed for longer than two months, it is recommended that either treatment is interrupted every eight weeks with a one-week break or dosage is reduced to the maintenance dose.

Restrictions on use

Those suffering from leukaemia or HIV should consult a healthcare professional before using Echinaforce.

Contra-indications

None known.

Pregnancy and nursing

No restrictions known.

Adverse reactions

None known.

Ingredients

Echinacea purpurea herb	95 per cent
Echinacea purpurea root	5 per cent

(Alcohol content: approximately 64 per cent)

Application

Bacterial infections (respiratory tract infections, urinary infections and skin infections); viral infections (influenza, herpes, chickenpox and ME); fungal infections (candida, ringworm and thrush); wound healing (cuts, post-operative care, varicose ulcers).

Mild, acute or chronic infections are a common occurrence. Echinacea taken internally can be very beneficial in these cases as it reduces the severity of symptoms and the duration of infections. This is achieved by stimulating the immune system, increasing the ability of the body to handle infections.

Echinacea may also be taken over a long-term period at a maintenance dose to increase the resistance to further infections.

The herb has also been shown to have the ability to improve the process of wound healing. It may be used both internally and externally (around the wound) for cuts, ulcers, burns, stings and infected or poorly healing superficial wounds.

❧ ELEUTHEROCOCCUS ❧

Description

The root of the herb *Eleutherococcus senticosus*, commonly referred to simply as Eleutherococcus, is an example of an 'adaptogen'. This has been defined as a substance which enables the body's metabolism to adapt and cope with unfavourable conditions such as physical and psychological stress, infections and environmental pollutants.

The plant is a tall prickly shrub, native to Eastern Asia and, particularly, Siberia. This gives rise to its common name Siberian ginseng, which is slightly misleading as it belongs to a totally different genus and is completely unrelated to *Panax ginseng*.

Mode of action

Adaptogenic activity; immune stimulant; supports the nervous system; enhances adrenal function; regulation of metabolism in tissues.

The adaptogenic action of Siberian ginseng is non-specific but appears to be an accumulation of the individual effects of a group of glycosides called eleutherosides.

The herb is able to support the body during periods of excessive physical and psychological stresses, as it acts directly on the adrenal–pituitary axis, increasing the body's resistance and its capacity to cope with these stresses. It contains enzymes, saponins and naturally occurring steroids which work together to support the metabolic processes of the body, giving a 'revitalising' effect.

Polysaccharides present in the root are responsible for stimulating the immune system, helping the body deal with chronic inflammatory and infective conditions by activating T-lymphocytes and the production of interferon.

Dosage information
ADULTS: 20–30 drops in a little water twice a day.
CHILDREN: May be used when appropriate at half the adult dose.

Duration of administration
There are no contra-indications to the long-term use of this herb. However, it is recommended that if Eleutherococcus is needed for longer than a period of two months, a two-week break from treatment is taken.

Restrictions on use
None known.

Contra-indications
Those who suffer from hypertension, anxiety and schizophrenia should consult a practitioner before using this product.

Pregnancy and nursing
It should not be used during pregnancy or breastfeeding.

Adverse reactions
Those on medicines for heart disorders, nervous disorders, diabetes and those taking the oral contraceptive pills or HRT should consult a practitioner before using Eleutherococcus.

It should not be taken together with stimulants such as caffeine. Vitamins B and C should not be taken at the same time as Siberian Ginseng as the excretion of these vitamins may be enhanced.

Ingredients
Eleutherococcus senticosus 100 per cent
(Alcohol content: approximately 49 per cent)

Application

Enhances physical and mental performance; physical stress; psychological stress; fatigue; ME; convalescence.

There are many causes of stress and fatigue. Most occur as a result of excessive demands on our physical and psychological reserves. The tonic effects on these two planes of our health is seen with Eleutherococcus; it improves physical performance, endurance, tolerance to stress and at the same time supports and enhances the body's own powers of restoration. This last action is of relevance when considering the body's ability to recover from a variety of illnesses such as infections, allergies, trauma and surgery.

These actions are even more important in conditions such as ME, chronic illness and convalescence from acute illnesses.

❦ EUPHRASIA ❦

Description

A single herbal preparation containing *Euphrasia officinalis*. As the common name, eyebright, suggests, Euphrasia is a phytotherapeutic remedy traditionally used for maintaining the health of the eyes.

The eyebright plant is a small annual native to Britain and Europe. It is commonly found in grasslands and woods, usually at higher altitudes. It grows to a height of about 30cm and bears pale lilac flowers.

Eyebright has been widely used in Europe as far back as the seventeenth century. It has a place in literature: in Milton's poem *Paradise Lost* the Archangel Michael used 'Euphrasy' to clear Adam's sight.

Mode of action

Astringent; anti-inflammatory; antiseptic; anticatarrhal.

Euphrasia officinalis contains a number of important constituents which include an iridoid, aucubin, caffeic acid and tannins. The tannins are astringents which help to dry up secretions and have the ability to relieve inflammatory conditions of the mucous membranes.

Euphrasia is indicated for a variety of conditions which affect the eyes, nose and sinuses. It is beneficial in conjunctivitis and blepharitis (inflammation of the eyelids) and catarrhal conditions of the sinuses and nasal passages such as sinusitis and hay fever. In addition, caffeic acid has an antiseptic action and aucubin has an anti-inflammatory action – properties which enhance the action of Euphrasia in these inflammatory conditions.

Dosage information
ADULTS: 20 drops taken internally in a little water twice a day.
MAINTENANCE: 20 drops once a day.
CHILDREN: Half adult amount.

Duration of administration
The maintenance dose may be taken for long periods of time for chronic conditions.

Restrictions on use
The preparation should not be used externally without the prior advice of a practitioner.

Contra-indications
None known.

Pregnancy and nursing
No restrictions known.

Adverse reactions
None known.

Ingredients
Euphrasia officinalis 100 per cent
(Alcohol content: approximately 66 per cent)

Application
Conjunctivitis; blepharitis (inflammation of the eyelids); hay fever (irritated, itchy eyes).

The eyes are delicate organs which are constantly exposed to the environment. They may easily become infected, irritated or inflamed.

Conjunctivitis is a common condition where the protective membrane of the eyes (known as conjunctiva) become inflamed. This may be caused by bacterial or viral infections, allergies (e.g. pollen, animal fur) or irritation from dust, smoke, pollutants and excessive glare.

In these conditions, the white of the eyes becomes inflamed. In an attempt to wash away the irritant, an increase in tear production takes place, giving a 'watery' eye. At the same time, the eye may feel 'gritty'. Bacterial infection causes the production of pus and a sticky eye. When bacterial infection affects the eyelids, the condition of blepharitis results.

❦ GINKGO BILOBA ❦

Description
This extract is made from the freshly harvested leaves of *Ginkgo biloba*. It possesses a number of common names. In China it is known as the 'memory tree', because of its action in maintaining and improving memory.

It is now generally accepted that the ginkgo tree is the world's oldest species of tree. Its medicinal use can be traced to the oldest Chinese *Materia Medica* dating back to around 3000 BC. Traditional Chinese medicine describes the ability of ginkgo leaves to 'benefit the brain'. Today, ginkgo extracts are among the most widely prescribed phytomedicines in both Germany and France. In Germany alone, ten million prescriptions for ginkgo are written each year, by more than 100,000 physicians.

Mode of action
Inhibits platelet aggregation; antioxidant; stabilises cell membranes; improves oxygen and glucose utilisation by the tissues; reduces arteriolar spasms.

There are a number of compounds which may be isolated from *Ginkgo biloba*. Terpenes account for about 6 per cent of ginkgo extracts and exist as ginkgolides and bilobalides. These substances increase arterial blood supply, especially to the brain, enhancing tissue utilisation of oxygen and glucose.

Effective brain function requires a large amount of energy, which is dependent on a constant supply of glucose and oxygen. If the circulation to the brain is impeded, a chain reaction is triggered which may eventually lead to cell and tissue damage and even death of these structures.

Ginkgolides inhibit a substance called PAF (platelet activating factor), which is responsible for platelet aggregation and clot formation. PAF is also involved in many inflammatory and allergic reactions which cause arteriolar spasm and reduce blood supply. This substance has also recently been implicated in acute asthmatic attacks and it has been suggested to some clinicians that ginkgo may be of benefit to asthmatics.

Other constituents of ginkgo which have significant action include the flavonoid compounds.

Cell membranes contain unsaturated fatty acids which are susceptible to attack by free radicals. Ginkgo has been found to have antioxidant activity, a free-radical scavenger, protecting cells from damage. Cells of the central nervous system are particularly vulnerable to the effects of free radicals, as they contain a higher proportion of cell membranes.

Ginkgo has been extensively studied in both laboratory and clinical trials. It is of great interest to note that the whole extract of the plant is more active than the individual components. This implies a high degree of synergism between the various chemical components, and supports one of the fundamental principles of phytotherapy.

Dosage information
ADULTS: 15 drops in a little water three times a day before meals.
CHILDREN: It is unlikely that this product will be needed in children without medical supervision.

Duration of administration
No restrictions on long-term usage known.

Restrictions on use
None known.

Contra-indications
None known.

Pregnancy and nursing
No restrictions known.

Adverse reactions
None known. However, it is best not taken alongside long-term low-dose aspirin.

Ingredients
Ginkgo biloba 100 per cent
(Alcohol content: approximately 61 per cent)

Application

Improvement of arterial circulation; cold hands and feet; chilblains; prevention and recovery from strokes; poor short-term memory; Raynaud's disease; senile dementia; tinnitus/dizziness; mastalgia (painful breasts).

An effective blood supply is vitally important for optimal tissue function. It is blood which transports oxygen and nutrients to the tissues and waste products away from them. Many conditions could arise as a result of an inadequate or interrupted blood supply. Amongst these are angina and heart attacks, transient ischaemic attacks and strokes, Raynaud's disease and intermittent claudication (poor circulation in the legs).

Mastalgia is an inflammatory condition, usually resulting from hormonal imbalances. Ginkgo has been found to be of help with these symptoms, probably mediated via its action on PAF.

🦋 DEVIL'S CLAW 🦋

Description

A herbal anti-inflammatory made from the tubers of *Harpagophytum procumbens*, a plant native to the southern parts of Africa.

It was formerly known as Harpagophytum, a term used to describe the branching, wood-like and barbed fruit which appear in the rainy season. It is the tubers or the storage roots of the plant, measuring approximately 20 cm in length, which are used medicinally. After collection, they are dried quickly to 90 per cent of the original fresh weight to prevent the growth of fungi on the surface of the tubers.

Mode of action

Anti-inflammatory; antirheumatic; analgesic; bitter tonic.

The anti-inflammatory, antirheumatic and analgesic properties of Devil's Claw are due to a group of components called iridoids, the principal of which is harpagoside.

This anti-inflammatory activity has been shown to be equivalent to that of corticosteroids, but without the side effects associated with these drugs even during long-term use (Weiss).

The corticosteroid-like activity makes the herb of benefit in autoimmune conditions. These are conditions where the body's immune system mounts a self-destructive attack on the cells of the body, giving rise to inflammation and swelling. There are many examples of autoimmune conditions which are frequently encountered, the most common of which are probably rheumatoid arthritis, lupus and some thyroid illnesses.

The action of Devil's Claw on the immune system and its cortiscosteroid-like activity gives the herb a role in the treatment of allergic and inflammatory conditions such as hay fever and urticaria.

Devil's Claw is also known as a bitter tonic, being able to stimulate the appetite, improving digestion and reducing flatulence. However, it is seldom employed in this role in modern phytotherapy.

Dosage information

ADULTS: 15 drops in a little water three times a day before meals.

CHILDREN: Half adult amount.

Duration of administration

For maximum benefit, it is likely that Devil's Claw will have to be used for several months.

Restrictions on use

None known. Whilst certain texts have stated that Devil's Claw is contra-indicated in diabetics, there appears to be no evidence to support this (Newell *et al*).

Pregnancy and nursing

It should not be taken during pregnancy without medical supervision.

Adverse reactions

None known.

Ingredients

Harpagophytum procumbens 100 per cent
(Alcohol content: approximately 53 per cent)

Application

Rheumatic conditions; painful/inflammatory conditions (muscular pain, sciatica, bursitis, gout and fibromyalgia); autoimmune conditions; allergies (hay fever).

Inflammation is a defensive response of the body to injury, which causes widening (dilation) of blood vessels with redness, pain, heat and swelling. The process involves the release of prostaglandins which stimulate pain receptors.

Devil's claw has been shown to be beneficial in acute and chronic conditions of the musculoskeletal system, where inflammation is present. It reduces pain and inflammation probably mediated through the corticosteroid-like action.

The ability for devil's claw to be of help in autoimmune conditions makes it useful in conditions such as rheumatoid arthritis (RA) and systemic lupus erythematosus (SLE).

Its action in stabilising the immune system gives it a role in the treatment of allergies such as hay fever.

❦ HAWTHORN–GARLIC COMPLEX ❦

Description
This preparation, formerly known as Arterioforce capsules, contains the fresh herbal extracts of garlic, hawthorn and passion flower combined with vitamin E. Hawthorn–Garlic Complex has been formulated to help with the heart and arterial circulation.

Mode of action
Lowers blood cholesterol levels; reduces platelet aggregation; vasodilator; antioxidant.

Garlic (*Allium sativum*) has now been shown to have a significant action in lowering the levels of cholesterol and triglycerides in the blood. At the same time it reduces the level of low density lipoproteins (LDL) while increasing the levels of high density lipoproteins (HDL).

It is now recognised that the ratio of HDL to LDL is a very significant factor in arterial disease. LDL carries cholesterol to the tissues, whereas HDL carries cholesterol back to the liver for metabolism and excretion. The relative amounts of HDL to LDL can thus determine whether cholesterol is broken down by the liver, or deposited in tissues. As the HDL to LDL ratio increases, platelet aggregation and plasma viscosity decrease, leading to improved blood flow and a reduced tendency for clot formation.

Garlic is also known to lower blood pressure and it possesses antioxidant activity, protecting cell membranes from being damaged by free radicals. Vitamin E is also a powerful antioxidant which supports the action of garlic.

Crataegus oxyacantha (hawthorn) contains procyanidins, which increase blood flow to the muscles of the heart and the extremities of the body through relaxation of the muscles in the wall of the arteries and arterioles. These substances also strengthen and stabilise the blood vessels, helping to prevent destructive changes taking place.

Dosage information
ADULTS: One or two capsules with a little water twice a day.
CHILDREN: It is unlikely that this product would be indicated for children.

Duration of administration
Hawthorn–Garlic Complex should be taken over a period of several months for its full effect. It is completely safe for long-term treatment. It is important not to discontinue a medically prescribed cardiovascular medication while taking the preparation.

Restrictions on use
None known.

Contra-indications
None known.

Pregnancy and nursing
Not recommended without medical advice.

Adverse reactions
None known. It may be taken alongside pharmaceutical medicines, but it would be best to seek the advice of a doctor or practitioner before doing so.

Ingredients
Allium sativa	150 mg
Crataegus oxyacantha	50 mg
Passiflora incarnata	20 mg
Vitamin E	15 mg
Beeswax	15 mg
Soya lecithin in a gelatin capsule	2.5 mg

Application
Conditions associated with arteriosclerosis (angina, intermittent claudication); high cholesterol levels; mild hypertension.

Arteriosclerosis is commonly referred to as hardening of the arteries. It is a progressive condition which may be found in any artery, although most commonly it is the circulation to the heart, the brain and the legs which are affected.

Arteriosclerosis starts with the deposition of fat and cholesterol in an artery. This initiates the formation of a 'plaque' which thickens the artery, giving rise to a loss of elasticity in the vessel wall and an increase in blood pressure. At the same time the blood vessels become narrowed, reducing blood flow to vital organs. As the plaque increases in size, blood flow is reduced further. At the same time, it encourages the formation of platelet clots.

Many of the major risk factors in arteriosclerosis – diet, stress, personality type, exercise and smoking are controllable. Other factors such as genetic tendency are not.

🦋 HYPERICUM 🦋

Description
A tincture prepared from *Hypericum perforatum* (St John's wort), which has had a traditional use as a 'mood elevator'. We now know that this herb has specific actions which influence the chemical neurotransmitters in the brain.

Mode of action
Antidepressant; antiviral; pain reliever; anti-inflammatory; promotes wound healing; antimicrobial.

It is not possible to assign the antidepressant effects of *Hypericum perforatum* to a specific constituent. The mechanism responsible for the antidepressant effect of *Hypericum perforatum* was once believed to be associated with monoamine oxidase inhibition (MAOI). Monoamine oxidase is an enzyme which breaks down amines found in the brain and the intestinal tract. The action of MAOI in depression is to increase the amount of amines in the brain. However, it is now thought that the level of MAO inhibition found in the plant extracts is not sufficient to account for its clinically proven antidepressant activity. Hypericin, which was thought to be the active constituent, has low MAOI activity while other constituents quercetin, luteolin and campherol are now known to have higher MAOI activity.

Hypericin is also able to increase levels of the neurotransmitter serotonin, which many now consider to be the main antidepressant mechanism found in Hypericum. Flavonoids and xanthones present have also been shown to inhibit the enzyme catechol-o-methyltransferase.

Whilst the precise action of the herb is still unclear, the benefits in depression have been clearly shown in numerous clinical trials, with improvements in symptoms such as tiredness, feelings of sadness, hopelessness, uselessness, emotional fear and disturbed sleep.

Taken internally, the flavonoids present in St John's wort have an analgesic action which can reduce pain in neuralgia, fibrositis and sciatica. These compounds have also been shown to possess activity against a number of viruses including the influenza virus and herpes simplex virus types 1 and 2.

Applied externally it is a valuable antibacterial, anti-inflammatory remedy which will aid in the healing of burns, wounds and infections.

Dosage information
ADULTS: 20 drops in a little water twice a day before meals.
CHILDREN: It is unlikely that this product would be indicated for children.

St John's wort does not potentiate the sedative effects of alcohol. It does not cause drowsiness so can be used when driving or operating machinery.
EXTERNAL USE: St John's wort oil may be applied to painful areas several times daily. The edges of small wounds may be dabbed with St John's wort oil two or three times a day.

Duration of administration
Clinical trials suggest that best results in depression are seen after four weeks of treatment.

Restrictions on use
Those using prescribed antidepressant medication should ideally seek medical advice before using the herb *Hypericum perforatum.*

Contra-indications
None known.

Pregnancy and nursing
Not recommended without medical supervision.

Adverse reactions
Exposure to the sun while taking *Hypericum perforatum* may result in a skin reaction. This is more common when Hypericum is applied externally.

Ingredients
Hypericum perforatum 100 per cent
(Alcohol content: approximately 63 per cent)

Application
Mild to moderate depression; seasonal affective disorder (SAD); viral infections.

Many people suffer from depression. It is estimated that, at any one time, 10–20 per cent of the population will experience these symptoms, with twice as many women than men being affected. Symptoms of depression include lowness of mood, lack of interest and enjoyment in usual activities, decreased energy levels, tiredness, sleep disturbances, poor concentration and altered appetite. A person is considered to be depressed when he or she experiences several symptoms of depression each day for a period of over two weeks.

Depression is now thought to be caused by lowered levels of certain chemical neurotransmitters in the brain. In recent studies *Hypericum perforatum* has been found to be beneficial in alleviating many symptoms associated with depression, when taken over a four-week period, without the side effects experienced with conventional antidepressant medication (see Appendix I).

❦ HYPERICUM COMPLEX ❦

Description
Hypericum Complex, formerly known as Hyperiforce, is a fresh herbal extract of *Hypericum perforatum, Melissa officinalis* and *Humulus lupulus*.

The herb Hypericum has been used for many years as an antidepressant. The combination of this with the anti-anxiety herbs, Melissa and Humulus, makes this Hypericum Complex particularly useful for those who suffer from depression which is accompanied by anxiety and restlessness.

Mode of action
Antidepressant; calming action.

Numerous clinical studies have shown St John's wort (*Hypericum perforatum*) to be effective in the treatment of depression. It is, however, still not possible to assign the antidepressant effects of this herb to specific constituents. Recent research indicates that it would seem unlikely that hypericins are the only active antidepressant principal, but that other flavonoids are involved in the action of the total extract. It has now been suggested that the action of Hypericum is mediated through the reduction in the number of serotonin receptors. Hypericum extracts have also been shown to possess antiviral and antimicrobial effects.

Lemon balm (*Melissa officinalis*) has a gentle sedative action, easing tension and anxiety. Nervous digestive disorders are relieved by its carminative, antispasmodic effects on the digestive system.

Hops (*Humulus lupulus*) have a sedative action which is helpful in insomnia. The calming action is also useful in tension states, such as irritable bowel syndrome (IBS).

In 1995, Hypericum Complex was the subject of a clinical trial in Switzerland. In a study by Pfister-Hotz *et al,* 74 per cent of patients with depression were found to have responded to treatment using this product, with the best improvement seen between two and four weeks after commencing treatment. The authors also found Hyperiforce (Hypericum Complex) to be 'very well tolerated'.

Dosage information
ADULTS: 30 drops in a little water two or three times a day.
CHILDREN: It is unlikely that Hypericum Complex will be indicated for children. (If a child requires support of the nervous system, *Avena sativa* should be used.)

Duration of administration
Clinical trials suggest that best results are seen with at least four weeks of treatment.

Restrictions on use
None known.

Contra-indications
A very few who use the herb *Hypericum perforatum* internally experience skin reactions. These reactions are more common

when Hypericum is applied externally to the skin. Skin reactions also depend on the presence of sunlight and hence are more common beyond the borders of the United Kingdom.

Pregnancy and nursing
It is not recommended during pregnancy.

Adverse reactions
None known.

Ingredients
Hypericum perforatum	65 per cent
Melissa officinalis	20 per cent
Humulus lupulus	15 per cent

(Alcohol content: approximately 61 per cent)

Application
Depression with anxiety and tension; mood swings associated with menopause; seasonally affective disorders.

In recent years, the incidence of depression has been on the increase. It is estimated that between 10 and 20 per cent of the population will suffer from this condition at some time during their lifetime. Women are more likely to be affected than men. Hopelessness, dejection, loss of self-esteem, difficulty in concentrating and sleep disturbance are some of the features associated with depression.

Hypericum perforatum, if taken over a longer period of time, has a beneficial effect on mild to moderate depressive states without the potential for addiction and with virtually no side effects (see Appendix I).

Depression seldom exists alone and the combination of anti-anxiety herbs in this preparation can be useful in practice.

Seasonally affective disorders are depressive disorders triggered by an imbalance in the neurotransmitters found in the brain, probably resulting from a lack of sunlight.

❧ IVY–THYME COMPLEX ❧

Description
This preparation, formerly known as Bronchosan, is a combination of herbs formulated to help soothe coughs which are associated with catarrh and other bronchial symptoms.

It is prepared from a number of herbs – common ivy, thyme, pimpernel, white horehound and liquorice. These herbs possess differing properties which, when combined, work synergistically, contributing to the overall efficacy of the preparation. Essential oils of anise and eucalyptus are added for flavouring.

Mode of action

Mucolytic action (thins mucus/catarrh); expectorant (expels catarrh); mild cough suppressant (anti-irritant); demulcent (soothing action).

Common ivy (*Hedera helix*) is an example of a herb which exerts an expectorant action on the respiratory tract of a reflex, irritative action on the stomach due to its saponin constituents. Expectorants encourage the loosening and elimination of mucus from the respiratory tract. These substances are beneficial in catarrhal conditions and chronic inflammatory bronchial disease. Ivy also has antispasmodic properties, helping to prevent and relieve coughing spasms.

The primary active components of thyme (*Thymus vulgaris*) are the volatile oils, especially thymol. These act locally on the lungs as they are eliminated from the body by the respiratory tract, disinfecting the airways, relaxing bronchial spasm and exerting a mucolytic action (decreases the viscosity of mucus). These actions are of benefit in bronchitis, hacking coughs and catarrh.

Pimpernel (*Pimpinella saxifraga*) is another herb with mucolytic action. In addition, it is an expectorant with anti-inflammatory activity, actions which are mediated by the saponins and volatile oils present.

The main active principal of white horehound (*Marrubium vulgare*) is the saponin, marrubiin. This substance stimulates secretions of the bronchial mucosa, an action which is enhanced by the presence of a volatile oil, making it a useful remedy for bronchitis.

Liquorice (*Glycyrrhiza glabra*) is an old favourite, added as much for its flavour as its medicinal action. Glycyrrhizin is a saponin which acts as an expectorant, whole another saponin, glycyrrhetinic acid, has a centrally active antitussive action, calming down the cough reflex. The flavonoids present help to reduce bronchial spasm.

Dosage information

ADULTS: 15 drops in a little water two or three times a day.
CHILDREN: Half adult dose.

Bronchosan may be used safely in children and diabetics – many cough mixtures contain sugar.

Duration of administration
No restrictions on long-term usage known.

Restrictions on use
Whilst Ivy–Thyme Complex is suitable for both acute and chronic bronchial conditions, it is not intended to be an anti-infective preparation. If infection is present, taking Echinaforce will support the immune system.

Avoid sunbathing while using this preparation, as Pimpinella may cause photosensitivity.

Pregnancy and nursing
Not recommended.

Adverse reactions
None known.

Ingredients
Hedera helix	30 per cent
Thymus vulgaris	25 per cent
Pimpinella saxifraga	25 per cent
Marrubium vulgare	10 per cent
Glycyrrhiza glabra	10 per cent

(Alcohol content: approximately 48 per cent)

Application
Infective coughs; acute bronchitis; chronic bronchitis and emphysema; bronchiectasis.

Coughs are distressing symptoms in many respiratory conditions. It is a normal reflex, being an attempt by the body to eliminate foreign objects from the respiratory tract. In practice, most coughs are caused by:
1. Bacterial or viral infections which, if severe, can lead to acute bronchitis.
2. The chronic cough which results from lung disease – for example, chronic bronchitis, emphysema and bronchiectasis. Careful questioning will ensure that no underlying serious condition (e.g. asthma) is overlooked.

Expectorants reduce the viscosity of mucus, loosening the irritant from the respiratory tract and aiding expulsion. The antitussive and antispasmodic actions help to prevent coughing spasms without cough suppression.

❧ KELP ❧

Description

Kelp contains the herb *Fucus vesiculosus* (kelp) in tablet form.

Kelp is a variety of seaweed known to botanists as the long-frond brown alga. It grows to lengths of up to 20 feet in the temperate parts of the Pacific and Atlantic Oceans.

In the past, fishermen and their families used the dried plant for fuel and food. However, apart from in Japan, the use of seaweed as a food has never become too popular and nowadays most of us do not have seaweed featured as part of our normal diet.

Kelp is rich in iodine. Goitres, caused by iodine deficiency, were common in the eighteenth century. However, physicians of the day noticed that those living along coasts rarely developed the problem, presumably as a result of a diet which had a greater proportion of seafood, shellfish and seaweed.

Mode of action

Source of iodine and minerals; increases metabolic rate; binds heavy metals and large molecules.

Kelp contains large amounts of iodine, bromine, trace elements and vitamin A; the main activity, however, lies with its iodine content. The body needs only a small amount (about 150mcg) of the mineral each day.

Iodine is an important component of thyroid hormones. The production and secretion of these hormones is controlled by a complex 'negative feedback' mechanism involving the hypothalamus, pituitary gland and a number of hormones. Increasing the iodine available to the body will increase the activity of the thyroid gland, increasing the body's general metabolism, which can then help with obesity, constipation (by improving blood flow and enhancing food breakdown) and increasing the motility in the digestive system.

Kelp also contains substances known as alginates. These molecules have the unique property of being able to absorb onto their surfaces heavy metals, radioactive substances and organic molecules such as cholesterol.

Dosage information
ADULTS: Two tablets twice a day before eating. Not to be taken before bedtime.
CHILDREN: It is unlikely that kelp will be indicated in children without medical supervision.

Duration of administration
Dosage should not be exceeded.

Restrictions on use
Kelp is not advised for anyone with high blood pressure, kidney disorders or thyroid conditions unless under medical supervision. It should not be taken by anyone with an allergy to iodine. It should be taken during the day because it stimulates the endocrine system, which tends to disturb sleep.

Contra-indications
Not to be taken with thyroxine tablets unless under medical supervision.

Pregnancy and nursing
Not recommended unless under medical supervision.

Adverse reactions
None known.

Ingredients
Each 250mg tablet contains:
Fucus vesiculosus   225mg
Excipients: lactose, glucose, Arabic gum, magnesium stearone.

Application
Stimulates metabolism; improves mental and physical alertness; detoxification.

Iodine is an essential element in thyroid function. Thyroid hormones regulate the growth and development of the body, nervous system activity and the rate of many metabolic processes. Some symptoms associated with low thyroid function are dry hair and skin, cold hands and feet, muscle weakness, rapid fatigue and a tendency to gain weight easily.

The main use of kelp is to increase the metabolic rate. In addition, its ability to bind to large molecules and heavy metals makes it useful as a detoxification agent. In the past, the US

Nuclear Regulatory Commission advised that three ounces of kelp a week be taken to reduce the absorption of strontium-90, in the event of radioactive accidents such as that seen at Chernobyl.

Kelp has also been shown to have the ability to reduce cholesterol levels by binding to this molecule in the digestive tract, before absorption into the blood.

❧ KNOTGRASS COMPLEX ❧

Description

Knotgrass Complex, previously known as Imperthritica, is one of Alfred Vogel's oldest formulations. It is a herbal combination formulated to improve and support the function of the musculoskeletal system. It is of benefit in relieving the symptoms associated with arthritic conditions by strengthening the soft tissue elements of joints. It also has a cleansing action on the joints and other parts of the body.

Mode of action

Rich in silica; strengthens soft tissue; cleansing/diuretic; anti-inflammatory.

Most of the herbs in this preparation have a degree of diuretic action. The increase in the volume of urine results in an increase in excretion of waste matter. This in turn eliminates unwanted toxic material from the soft tissues of the body.

Betula alba (birch) contains saponins and flavonoids which have anti-inflammatory activity. It is also a bitter digestive stimulant and diuretic, a combination which is useful in alleviating inflammatory conditions such as rheumatism and arthritis.

Solidago virgaurea (golden rod) is a diuretic which also possesses anti-inflammatory action.

Urtica dioica (nettle) increases the excretion of uric acid and other acid metabolites from the body. It also contains nutrients which are important for the soft tissues of joints, especially silica.

Silica is also present in *Polygonum aviculare* (knotgrass) and *Equisetum arvense* (horsetail). Silica-rich plants assist the immune system in cleansing the body of toxins. An improvement in the elasticity and strength of connective tissue is also seen.

Interestingly, it is now thought that crystalline deposits in joints may be responsible for many cases of arthritis. The dynamics of the joint are altered, leading to inflammation. Improving the elimination and cleansing of body fluids removes the end products of metabolism from tissues together with accumulated toxins which are known to cause and aggravate arthritis and rheumatism.

Dosage information
ADULTS: 15–20 drops in a little water twice a day before meals.
CHILDREN: Half adult amount.

Duration of administration
There are no restrictions on long-term usage.

Restrictions on use
None known.

Pregnancy and nursing
None known.

Adverse reactions
None known.

Ingredients

Solidago virgaurea	23 per cent
Potentilla tormentilla	11 per cent
Iva moschata	11 per cent
Mentha piperita	6 per cent
Polygonum aviculare	16 per cent
Urtica dioica	11 per cent
Betula alba	11 per cent
Equisetum arvense	11 per cent

(Alcohol content: approximately 55 per cent)

Application
Osteoarthritis; rheumatoid arthritis; lower back pain (lumbago); gout; carpal tunnel syndrome.

There are many forms of arthritis but the main ones commonly seen are osteoarthritis and rheumatoid arthritis. There are a number of features which differentiate them. Osteoarthritis is due to wear and tear of the joint. It mainly affects single, weight-bearing joints in the body, tending to be worse after use and is equally common in men and women. Rheumatoid arthritis is a chronic inflammatory disorder which can affect the whole body. Joints in the hands, feet, wrists, ankles and knees are mainly affected, most often occurring with a symmetrical distribution (i.e. both hands, both feet) and is more common in females.

Knotgrass Complex is helpful in both these complaints by reducing inflammation and eliminating toxins in the blood and soft tissues. It is of use in gout as the elimination of uric acid is improved.

❦ LINOFORCE ❦

Description
Linoforce is a laxative combining the gentle bulking action of linseed with the stimulating effects of senna leaves and *Rhamnus frangula*. It is formulated to help relieve occasional constipation or more long-standing conditions, arising from a 'lazy' bowel.

Mode of action
Bulk laxative; lubricant; bowel stimulant.

Linseed comes from the plant common flax (*Linum usitatissimum*). It contains 5–6 per cent mucilage, 30–40 per cent oil and 20 per cent protein.

The most important use for linseed is as a bulking agent. The mucilage which is present swells in the presence of water, endowing the seeds with tremendous 'bulking' ability. This action does not irritate the bowel but acts by increasing the 'fibre' content, mechanically filling the bowel and making the stools more voluminous. This in turn stops the stools from becoming dry and hard, reducing the absorption of toxins. The oils present in linseed act as a lubricant, supporting the bulking action. Linseed is usually effective after 12–24 hours, reaching a maximum after several days. It must be taken with plenty of fluid to allow the seeds to swell and exert their action.

Both senna (*Cassia*) and frangula (alder buckthorn bark) act through the activity of anthraquinone glycosides. These substances are poorly absorbed from the small intestine but are converted (hydrolysed) by the bacteria of the large intestine into the active substance known as aglycone. This exerts a laxative effect on the colon by increasing colonic motility, reducing transit time and absorption of water from stools.

Dosage information

ADULTS: One to two teaspoonfuls to be taken in the morning with about 200ml of water.

CHILDREN: If appropriate, half the adult amount can be given.

Linoforce can be sprinkled on breakfast cereals. However, plenty of fluid should be taken with the preparation. If a further dose is required, then one to two teaspoonfuls can be taken in the evening.

Duration of administration

Ideally, Linoforce should be taken only for as long as necessary. Generally, it is not advisable to take laxatives on a long-term basis. However, there are some who need a constant regular dosage of laxative agents, to ensure a degree of bowel movement. Whilst this is not ideal, there are no specific contra-indications to using Linoforce in this manner.

Restrictions on use

Not to be used, unless under medical supervision, if constipation is caused by tension, colitis, intestinal obstruction and conditions with accompanying abdominal pain, nausea, fever, vomiting or diarrhoea.

Contra-indications

See above.

Pregnancy and nursing

Should be avoided during pregnancy and lactation.

Adverse reactions

If abdominal cramping occurs, dosage should be reduced.

Ingredients

Linseed	43.03 per cent
Sennae folium	12.91 per cent
Rhamnus frangula cortex	1.07 per cent
Crystallised sucrose	12.05 per cent
Vanilla	0.02 per cent
Ginger essence	0.02 per cent
(Excipients to 100g)	

Application

Constipation; regulation of bowel movements.

Constipation is a problem which we can all experience at one time or another. It is defined as the infrequent passage of hard, dry motions and most commonly arises through lack of fibre in the diet and an inadequate fluid intake. Constipation may also arise as a result of lack of exercise, as a side effect of drugs (e.g. codeine in painkillers) and certain antidepressants. The problem is usually more predominant in the elderly, those who are inactive and during pregnancy.

Strong laxatives are sometimes abused, being taken regularly on a long-term basis. This can cause harm as the bowel is constantly irritated with prolonged use, leading to a distended and 'lazy' bowel.

The predominant ingredient of Linoforce is linseed, which has a gentle bulking action, increasing the frequency and quantity of bowel movement. This is combined with small amounts of the stimulant laxatives which accelerate this bulking action.

❧ MENOSAN ❧

Description
Menosan is prepared from the fresh leaves of sage (*Salvia officinalis*).

Salvia officinalis is one of our oldest medicinal plants. The Greeks and Romans first used it as a preservative for meat. It was believed that, amongst other actions, it could improve the memory and presumably increase wisdom – a term which probably gave us the origin of the common name, sage. This has greater relevance in that the herb has recently been investigated for its use in Alzheimer's disease.

Sage contains volatile oils, tannins and flavonoids. In the past, it has been used for a wide variety of conditions. Nowadays its prime role is as a useful remedy for alleviating excessive sweating and menopausal hot flushes.

Mode of action
Phyto-oestrogen; oestrogen action; hypothalmic action; antiseptic; astringent.

Sage has been found to be beneficial in reducing the frequency and severity of hot flushes and night sweats which accompany the menopause because it contains phyto-oestrogens. These substances are capable of binding to oestrogen receptors on cells, exerting a mild oestrogenic effect, which helps to correct the lower oestrogen levels which occur at this time of life.

At around the time of the menopause, the amount of oestrogen produced by the ovaries begins to diminish. The lower levels of hormones in the blood trigger the release of a specific regulating factor from the hypothalamus in the brain, encouraging more hormone production from the ovaries. At the same time, the hypothalamus is also the control centre for temperature regulation. It is an important intermediary between the nervous system and endocrine system. Many of the physical and mental symptoms which occur during menopause are a result of an imbalance in this control mechanism.

The volatile oils (especially thujone) in sage are good antiseptics. Tannins are anti-inflammatory and astringent and this combination is useful for throat and mouth infections and inflammation, especially when used as a gargle.

Taken internally, sage can reduce the secretion of saliva and breast milk. This latter application is useful in weaning infants off breast milk.

Dosage information
ADULTS: 15–20 drops in a little water three times a day before meals. If night sweats are particularly severe, 30 drops should be taken before bedtime.

AS A GARGLE: Ten drops of salvia tincture in half a cup of hot water to be used four to six times daily as needed, for sore throats.

CHILDREN: It is not likely that this product will be indicated internally for children.

Duration of administration
No restrictions known.

Restrictions on use
Those who suffer from diabetes and epilepsy should consult a practitioner before using sage. In the past, authors have suggested that sage is contra-indicated in hypertension but more modern texts have not supported this.

Pregnancy and nursing
It should not be used in pregnancy or breastfeeding.

Adverse reactions
None known.

Ingredients
Salvia officinalis 100 per cent
(Alcohol content: approximately 60 per cent)

Application
Hot flushes; excessive sweating (hyperhidrosis); stops breast milk production; excessive salivation; inflammation/ulceration of mouth and throat.

The menopause signals the end of the reproductive life of a woman. This usually occurs between the ages of 45 and 60, although it may start in the middle to late thirties. Menopause is a time of fundamental hormonal and functional adjustment and many of the distressing symptoms, such as hot flushes, mood changes, insomnia, palpitations, vaginal soreness and cystitis, are the result of the body trying to adapt to these changes.

Sage is a phyto-oestrogen but does not contain any oestrogenic molecules. Its action depends on the ability to trigger off oestrogen production by oestrogen-producing cells and its oestrogen effects when binding to oestrogen receptors.

Its direct antibacterial action is useful for inflammation of the mouth and throat, which is related to infections.

❦ MILK THISTLE COMPLEX ❦

Description
Milk Thistle Complex, formerly known as Boldocynara, is a tincture prepared by combining a number of 'liver herbs'. It is a traditional herbal liver tonic which strengthens, cleanses and protects the liver. The major herbs used are artichoke, milk thistle and dandelion. Boldo and peppermint are added to support their actions.

Mode of action
Cholagogue with choleretic action; digestive stimulant.

Phytotherapists use herbs with cholagogue, choleretic and bitter properties to enhance liver and gallbladder function. Choleretics stimulate the production of bile from the liver; cholagogues increase the release of bile from the gallbladder; and bitters are digestive stimulants, improving digestive function. Breakdown and absorption of nutrients is enhanced, with an increase in the flow of digestive juices in the liver, stomach and pancreas.

Artichoke, dandelion, boldo and peppermint have all demonstrated cholagogue and choleretic action. In addition, they possess detoxifying and restorative properties which are necessary for improving liver function.

Globe artichoke (*Cynara scolymus*) reduces cholesterol and lipid levels in the blood through its action on the liver. A group of compounds called phenolic acids possess a protective and restorative function in the liver.

Silymarin, the main constituent of milk thistle (*Silybum marianum*) acts directly on the cell membranes of the liver, preventing cell damage and encouraging the regeneration of liver cells.

Dandelion (*Taraxacum officinale*) has a long history of traditional use in the treatment of liver and gallbladder problems. It is a diuretic and mild laxative, rich in minerals and nutrients. These features combine to make it an excellent cleansing agent.

Boldo and peppermint are spasmolytic, acting locally to produce smooth muscle relaxation which in turn helps to relieve stomach and intestinal colic as well as dyspepsia. Peppermint also has a carminative effect, largely due to the volatile oil content which is beneficial in reducing flatulence.

Dosage information

ADULTS: 15–20 drops in a little water twice a day after meals.
CHILDREN: Five drops in a little water twice a day after meals.

Ideally, this tincture should be held briefly in the mouth before swallowing to promote the bitter action of the herbs.

Duration of administration

No restrictions on long-term usage known.

Restrictions on use

None known.

Contra-indications

Medical opinion should be sought with acute and severe liver complaints such as hepatitis and biliary tract occlusion. This preparation may be used during the recovery from hepatitis, alcoholism, drugs and for gallbladder disease.

Pregnancy and nursing
Do not take if breastfeeding, as artichoke may interfere with milk production.

Adverse reactions
Increased frequency of bowel movements may occur because of the increased secretion of the digestive juices. If this happens, the dosage should be reduced.

Ingredients
Cynara scolymus	46 per cent
Silybum marianum	32 per cent
Taraxacum officinalis	12 per cent
Peumus boldus	7 per cent
Mentha piperita	3 per cent

(Alcohol content: approximately 63 per cent)

Application
Liver and gallbladder problems (jaundice, gallstones); to stimulate bile production (nausea/indigestion after eating fatty foods); digestive insufficiency (constipation, loss of appetite); high blood cholesterol; detoxification (alcohol abuse, long-term use of painkillers).

The liver performs many vital functions in the body. It stores vitamins and minerals, produces bile which is required for the breakdown of fat, and is the main organ involved in the metabolism of food, drugs and hormones.

Liver impairment can produce liver and gallbladder complaints and digestive disturbances. It is now well established that the 'liver herbs' can play an important role in restoring physiological function in these conditions.

The combination of artichoke and milk thistle is synergistic, enhancing the efficacy of the preparation. The ability of artichoke to lower cholesterol levels is of great use therapeutically.

❦ MOLKOSAN ❦

Description
The name Molkosan is derived from *molke*, the German word for whey. It is a naturally lacto-fermented whey which is concentrated during processing to ensure a high content of minerals, especially calcium, potassium, phosphorus and L(+) lactic acid. L(+) lactic acid gives the product a pH of 2.7 (very

acidic) which combines with its antiseptic action to inhibit bacterial and fungal infections. The lactose in Molkosan is present in its natural form, which does not cause digestive problems for lactose-intolerant or lactose-sensitive people.

Mode of action

Lowered pH (2.7) increases acidity; digestive enzyme stimulant; normalises intestinal flora; anti-infective (both internally and externally).

The low acidity created by Molkosan promotes the growth of normal digestive tract flora. It also normalises intestinal flora that has been disturbed.

Molkosan has been found to have antifungal activity. It can be applied directly to areas affected by fungal infection such as athlete's foot, ringworm and thrush. Solutions of Molkosan in water are also effective against a variety of scalp complaints such as dandruff and as a gargle it can be used for sore throats associated with oral thrush or bacterial infection.

Molkosan contains orotic acid, which is essential for the formation of DNA and RNA – the protein-building blocks of the body. Orotic acid combines with minerals to form orotates, which are easily absorbed by the body, acting as chemical buffers. These compounds help to create a beneficial environment which is important to health. It is especially useful in a slimming programme, as fat metabolism creates breakdown products which need to be buffered or neutralised.

As a slimming aid, Molkosan should be diluted 15ml to 100ml of mineral water or diluted vegetable juice for maximum benefit.

Dosage information

INTERNAL USE: One teaspoonful of Molkosan to a glass of mineral water taken internally three times a day before or with meals.

EXTERNAL USE: Apply to small wounds, abrasions and skin rashes, either neat or diluted to a ratio of 1:4 with water.

FOR INSECT BITES: Apply undiluted on the bite.

AS A GARGLE: Mix one tablespoonful of Molkosan with four tablespoonfuls of water and gargle.

AS HAIR AND BODY RINSE: Dilute Molkosan 1:10 with water and use this mixture to rinse hair and skin after showers. Do not rinse again with fresh water.

Duration of administration
No restrictions known.

Restrictions on use
None known.

Contra-indications
None known.

Pregnancy and nursing
No contra-indications known.

Adverse reactions
None known.

Ingredients
Fermented and Concentrated Milk Whey containing:

Total lactic acid	8,500mg
L(+) lactic acid	7,000mg
Lactose	4,000mg
Total minerals	1,000mg
Calcium	130mg
Potassium	190mg
Phosphorus	100mg
Magnesium	trace
Zinc	trace
Iron	trace
Chloride	trace
Orotic acid	trace
Vitamin B complex	trace
Vitamin C	trace

(Fat- and protein-free
50 kcal per 100g
 8 kcal per tablespoonful)

Application
Maintains healthy intestinal flora; antifungal (thrush, athlete's foot, ringworm); antibacterial; slimming aid.

The yeast *Candida albicans* is present in every individual. It normally lives harmlessly in the gastrointestinal tract.

Antibiotics are often responsible for upsetting the balance of the intestinal flora by suppressing the normal intestinal bacteria. This provides an opportunity for candidal overgrowth. The antifungal activity of Molkosan is due to its acidity and buffering capability. It is able to re-establish the normal balance of organisms in the digestive tract.

This antifungal activity is also useful topically against vaginal thrush, athlete's foot and ringworm. As a gargle, it is an effective remedy for sore throats, caused by either yeast or bacterial organisms.

The ability of orotic acid to enhance the digestive and metabolic processes make Molkosan useful as an aid to a calorie-controlled slimming programme.

❦ SAW PALMETTO COMPLEX ❦

Description
Saw Palmetto Complex was previously known as Prostasan. The main active constituent is saw palmetto fruit, which has a proven action on the prostate gland. This herb is now considered to be the prime remedy for prostate problems.

Saw palmetto is a herb which has a number of different botanical names. For many years it was known as *Sabal serrulata*. More recently, however, new botanical nomenclature has provided it with the name *Serenoa repens*.

The saw palmetto is a small palm with fan-shaped leaves. The fruit are dark red and the size of olives. It contains a volatile oil known as palmetto oil, which is one of the main active ingredients.

Mode of action
Inhibits hormone metabolism; anti-inflammatory; antiseptic.

The male testes secrete testosterone. This is converted within the prostate by the enzyme 5-alpha reductase to dihydrotestosterone (DHT). The enzyme 3-ketosteroid reductase enhances the binding of DHT to androgen receptors in the gland, causing the prostatic cells to enlarge, which in turn causes the whole gland to increase in size (hypertrophy). This is the condition known commonly as an enlarged prostate and referred to medically as benign prostatic hypertrophy (BPH).

Saw palmetto inhibits the enzyme 5-alpha reductase, which in turn reduces the amount of DHT produced. It also inhibits the binding of this compound by 3-kerosteroid reductase to the receptors. The result of all this is to alleviate congestion and inflammation in the prostate by inhibiting the production of inflammatory substances and their subsequent leakage through the capillaries into the surrounding tissue, thereby relieving symptoms associated with BPH.

Saw palmetto acts specifically on the prostate gland and does not affect androgen activity in other organs such as the testes.

Solidago virgaurea (golden rod) is a diuretic with important anti-inflammatory and antiseptic action which soothes urinary tract infections.

Echinacea purpurea (echinacea) has generalised immune stimulant, anti-inflammatory and antimicrobial properties which can help fight infection which may be present.

Populus tremula (white poplar bark) is a herb with mild analgesic properties which relieves pain and inflammation in urinary tract spasms and painful urination.

Dosage information
ADULTS: 10–20 drops in a little water two or three times a day.
MAINTENANCE: If symptoms are stable, a dose of 20 drops once
 a day will be appropriate.
CHILDREN: It is unlikely that this product will be indicated in
 children.

Duration of administration
There are no known restrictions on the length of treatment.

Restrictions on use
Medical advice should be sought if the condition persists or is accompanied by bleeding or a fever.

Pregnancy and nursing
Not applicable.

Adverse reactions
Men taking prescribed medicines for hormone adjustment should first consult their medical practitioner before using Saw Palmetto Complex.

Ingredients
Sabal serrulata fruct.	93.5 per cent
Solidago virgaurea	3.0 per cent
Echinacea purpurea herba	2.0 per cent
Populus tremulus	1.5 per cent

(Alcohol content: approximately 60 per cent)

Application
Prostate enlargement (BPH); cystitis in men secondary to BPH; prostatitis.

The prostate is a doughnut-shaped gland about the size of a chestnut and is part of the male reproductive system. The gland surrounds the urethra which carries urine flow from the bladder.

In older men, particularly those over 50, enlargement of the prostate may occur – a condition known as benign prostatic hypertrophy (BPH). The cause of this enlargement is an increased sensitivity of the prostatic cells to the levels of testosterone circulating in the body. BPH causes a disturbance to the flow of urine, resulting in frequent urination, particularly in the middle of the night (a condition known as nocturia), poor or painful urine flow and dribbling.

Prostatitis is a totally different condition of the prostate. It is seen most frequently in younger men, and is the result of infection, usually by bacteria, of the substance of the gland. The anti-inflammatory action of saw palmetto has some value in this condition.

🦋 SOLIDAGO COMPLEX 🦋

Description
This preparation, formerly known as Nephrosolid, is a combination of four freshly harvested herbal extracts. Its main constituent, *Solidago virgaurea*, is combined with *Betula pendula*, *Ononis spinosa* and *Equisetum arvense*. Solidago Complex is a kidney tonic. It has a diuretic action and is generally supportive to the kidneys.

Mode of action
Diuretic; anti-inflammatory; astringent; antiseptic.

Solidago virgaurea (golden rod) is a diuretic with important anti-inflammatory, antispasmodic and antiseptic action. It soothes irritations in the urinary tract caused by infections such as cystitis and urethritis, and prevents the formation and facilitates elimination of kidney stones.

Solidago virgaurea, *Equisetum arvense* (horsetail), *Betula pendula* (birch) and *Ononis spinosa* (spiny rest harrow) contains saponins, flavonoids and tannins. Their diuretic action is the result of the saponins and flavonoids. Saponins are also anti-inflammatory and tannins are astringent. This combined action makes Solidago Complex useful for keeping mild urinary tract infections in check, minimising damage to the walls of the ureters, bladder and urethra.

Diluting the urine prevents the crystallisation of insoluble salts which result in kidney stone formation, and the diuretic action flushes out any deposits already formed.

Equisetum arvense has a high mineral content. It contains especially high amounts of silica, which helps to heal and strengthen damaged tissue.

Dosage information
ADULTS: 10–15 drops in a little water three times a day.
CHILDREN: Half adult amount.

Duration of administration
No restrictions known.

Restrictions on use
If the urinary tract condition persists, or if there is nausea, vomiting, fever or blood in the urine, which could indicate a more serious problem, a medical practitioner should be consulted.

The preparation should not be taken as a diuretic for fluid retention associated with heart disorders or high blood pressure without prior medical advice.

Pregnancy and nursing
It may be used for cystitis during pregnancy.

Adverse reactions
None known.

Ingredients
Solidago virgaurea	69 per cent
Betula pendula	18 per cent
Ononis spinosa	7 per cent
Equisetum arvense	6 per cent

(Alcohol content: approximately 58 per cent)

Application
Kidney tonic; kidney stones; minor kidney and bladder inflammation.

The main function of the kidneys is the elimination of waste products from the body. This is achieved through the formation of urine, which also maintains a chemical balance in cells and tissues, regulating fluid balance and blood pressure. The anti-inflammatory and astringent properties of the herbs in Solidago Complex are useful in combating infection in the urinary tract.

Herbal diuretics can also be helpful in alleviating many urinary disorders such as infection and inflammation. Diluting the urine reduces the concentration of irritating and infective organisms present. In addition, increasing the flow of urine can help to dissolve or 'wash out' stones which are present in the urinary tract.

❦ TORMENTIL COMPLEX ❦

Description
Tormentil Complex, previously known as Tormentavena, is a combination of the fresh extracts of tormentil and oats. The main ingredient, tormentil, is a prime remedy in gastrointestinal disturbances where diarrhoea with accompanying inflammation and irritation are prominent.

The herb tormentil is a member of the rose family. It is found all over Europe in woods, moors and grassy pieces of ground. It is a small plant with yellow flowers and a thick root. The cross section of the root is red, giving rise to the common name 'bloodroot'.

Mode of action
Anti-diarrhoea; anti-inflammatory; antispasmodic; normalises bowel movement.

Potentilla tormentilla (tormentil) has a high tannin content (10–30 per cent), which is responsible for its astringent action on the digestive tract. Tannins bind to the proteins present in the mucous membranes, producing a coat on the membrane surface which protects the exposed tissues against irritation. This has the ability to form a barrier against most infective organisms and many toxins, slows down the frequency of bowel movements and encourages the healing of the affected bowel.

Avena sativa (oats) enhances the action of the remedy by exerting a mild sedative and restorative effect on the nervous system, which also calms an overactive digestive system. This is particularly relevant in the condition of irritable bowel syndrome.

Dosage information
ADULTS: 20–30 drops in a little water two or three times a day.
CHILDREN: Half adult amount.

Duration of administration
This is dependent on the underlying cause of the problem. No restrictions on long-term use known.

Restrictions on use
Medical advice should be sought if acute symptoms do not improve within 24–36 hours or if these are violent and accompanied by severe pain, vomiting, fever or blood loss. Babies and younger children may need special attention as they can easily become dehydrated.

Contra-indications
None known.

Pregnancy and nursing
None known. However, if diarrhoea persists for more than 24 hours in a pregnant woman, medical advice should be sought.

Adverse reactions
None known.

Ingredients
Potentilla tormentilla	75 per cent
Avena sativa	25 per cent

(Alcohol content: approximately 60 per cent)

Application
Diarrhoea; irritable bowel syndrome (with diarrhoea, alternating diarrhoea and constipation); diverticulitis; colitis; Crohn's disease.

Diarrhoea is the body's attempt to expel an irritant from the bowel. Infection and food poisoning cause inflammation in the gastrointestinal tract, resulting in diarrhoea and vomiting.

A number of antibiotics can upset the balance of the natural flora of the gut, giving rise to diarrhoea. It may also be a symptom of colitis, Crohn's disease and irritable bowel syndrome. Stress may be a significant factor, causing over-stimulation of the bowel, whereas chronic diarrhoea may be a sign of food allergy often related to dairy products or wheat.

Tannins exert an 'astringent' action on the bowel. This helps to relieve inflammatory bowel conditions and reduce the frequency and severity of loose motions.

❦ URTICA DIOICA ❦

Description
A fresh herbal extract of *Urtica dioica* (stinging nettle), which is considered by phytotherapists to be an excellent 'blood tonic', being able to provide nutritional support to the body.

Mode of action
Diuretic; nutritive blood tonic; lowers blood glucose levels; astringent; herbal antihistamine; increases breast milk production.

Urtica dioica (nettle) contains flavonoids, which account for its action as a diuretic. It increases excretion of chlorides, uric acid and other acid metabolites from the body, which may help to alleviate the symptoms associated with gout and arthritic conditions. This cleansing action is of value in chronic skin conditions, especially the itchy complaints such as eczema and nettle rash, where it also appears to posssess an anti-allergic action.

Nettle is a nutritive herb high in chlorophyll, vitamin C, iron, calcium potassium and silica. It has a restorative action in iron deficiency, anaemia and other deficiency conditions. Nettle also has a traditional use as a galactagogue – a herb which stimulates milk production in a nursing mother.

A mild blood sugar lowering action has been attributed to a glucoquinone present and this compound has been given the name urticin. The tannin content provides astringency both internally and externally and its haemostatic action slows down or stops any bleeding.

Dosage information
ADULTS: 20 drops in a little water twice a day before meals.
CHILDREN: Half the adult amount.

Duration of administration
Excessive use may interact with concurrent treatment for diabetes, high or low blood pressure.

Restrictions on use
None known.

Contra-indications
None known.

Pregnancy and nursing
It should be avoided in pregnancy. Use during lactation may stimulate milk production.

Adverse reactions
Rarely, allergic reactions have been observed. Gastrointestinal irritation has been documented in a few cases.

Ingredients
Urtica dioica 100 per cent
(Alcohol content: approximately 51 per cent)

Application
Detoxifier; gout; rheumatism/arthritis; iron deficiency anaemia; chronic skin disorders (e.g. eczema); allergies (e.g. hay fever, urticaria).

An acute attack of gout occurs as a result of uric acid crystals being deposited in joints. This occurs most predominantly at the base of the big toe, but gout can affect any joint of the body. White blood cells ingest these crystalline deposits, releasing enzymes which then cause inflammation. The detoxifying and cleansing action of Urtica eliminates the crystals. This same mechanism is used to explain the benefits of using Urtica in those with rheumatism and arthritis.

Its antihistamine action is of benefit in skin conditions such as eczema, where itch may be a predominant symptom. This action is particularly relevant in the allergic conditions such as urticaria and also hay fever.

❧ URTICALCIN ❧

Description
Urticalcin is a homoeopathic preparation containing *Urtica dioica*, calcium and silica. It is especially useful where a lack of calcium is present.

Mode of action
Source of calcium and silica; promotes calcium absorption; increases excretion of acidic compounds.

Urticalcin combines the herb *Urtica dioica* (stinging nettle) with the tissue salts *Silicea, Calcarea carbonica, Calcarea phosphorica* and *Natrium phosphorica.*

Urtica dioica (stinging nettle) is nutritive through its content of calcium, silica, potassium, iron, chlorophyll and vitamin C. It also has a diuretic action, helping to eliminate waste products from the body.

Silicea (silica) is an essential component of collagen which is present in connective tissue. It is found in large amounts in skin, hair, nails, bones, tendons and lymph nodes. It is also found in areas of active bone mineralisation, which suggests an association between silica and calcium binding in bones.

Both *Calcarea carbonica* (calcium carbonate) and *Calcarea phosphorica* (calcium phosphate) are easily absorbed sources of calcium, which is necessary for bone formation and proper nerve and muscle function. Calcium phosphate is present in all bones and will help in the healing of fractures, aiding tooth development in children.

Natrium phosphorica (sodium phosphate) influences cellular metabolism. It helps to maintain the correct acid-base balance in the cells promoting optimal function.

A Swiss study involving over 6,000 people showed that Urticalcin was very beneficial in the following conditions: strengthening fingernails, preventing tooth cavities, hair growth problems, fatigue, slow-healing wounds, recovery after bone fractures, prevention of colds and influenza, recovery after illness.

Dosage information
ADULTS: Three tablets twice a day. Allow to dissolve slowly under the tongue.
CHILDREN: Half adult amount.

Duration of administration
For maximum benefit the tablets should be taken for at least two months.

Restrictions on use
None known.

Contra-indications
None known.

Pregnancy and nursing
No restrictions known.

Adverse reactions
None known.

Ingredients

Urtica 1x	10.0mg
Silica 6x	2.5mg
Calcium carbonate 4x	0.5mg
Calcium phosphate 6x	0.5mg
Sodium phosphate 6x	0.5mg
(Excipients to 100mg)	

Application
Strengthens bones and nails; improves quality and appearance of hair; prevents bone loss in the elderly; aids recovery after bone fractures; enhances wound healing; improves teeth development in children.

Calcium is the most abundant mineral in the body. Ninety-nine per cent is found in bones and teeth while the remaining one per cent is used in nerve transmission, muscle contraction, blood clotting and enzyme activity.

Osteoporosis, muscle cramps, sleeplessness, increased nervousness and a tingling sensation in the arms can result from calcium deficiency. Bone constantly needs essential nutrients, especially calcium for healthy growth, development and maintenance.

Bone mass reaches a peak between the age of 35 and 40, then starts to decline because bone resorption is greater than bone formation. The loss in women after the menopause is greater because of oestrogen deficiency, which favours bone breakdown. Calcium requirements increase during pregnancy and lactation.

❧ UVA-URSI COMPLEX ❧

Description
This preparation, formerly known as Cystoforce, is a combination of herbs formulated by Alfred Vogel to relieve the symptoms associated with urinary tract infections. The main herbs of this remedy are *Arctostaphylos uva-ursi* (often just known as *uva-ursi*) and *Echinacea purpurea*.

Mode of action
Antiseptic; astringent; anti-inflammatory.

Arctostaphylos uva-ursi (bearberry) has antiseptic properties by virtue of a glycoside known as arbutin. This substance is absorbed from the gastrointestinal tract and passed into the bloodstream. It is then excreted by the kidneys unchanged into the urine. In the urine, arbutin is hydrolysed, splitting into glucose and a substance called hydroquinone. It is hydroquinone which possesses a direct antiseptic action in the kidneys, ureter and, particularly, the bladder. This conversion is encouraged if the urine is alkaline.

The high tannin content of *uva-ursi* has a significant astringent effect upon the membranes of the urinary tract. This strengthening and toning action is beneficial in some forms of bedwetting and incontinence.

Echinacea purpurea has indirect anti-infective properties, stimulating white blood cell proliferation and interferon activity.

The volatile oil component of *Achillea millefolium* (yarrow) is a diuretic and urinary antiseptic, which is beneficial for urinary tract infections.

Rhus aromatica (sweet sumach) is known for its astringency (due to its tannin component) and is especially indicated for urinary incontinence and bedwetting in young people.

Dosage information
GENERALLY: 15 drops in a little water twice a day.
ACUTE SITUATIONS: 20 drops in a little water three times a day.
MAINTENANCE: 15 drops once a day.
CHILDREN: Half the adult amount.

The hydrolysis of arbutin, which produces hydroquinone, takes place most easily in an alkaline environment. It is thus best to avoid high-protein foods, tea, coffee and alcohol, whilst increasing fruit (apart from citrus fruit) and vegetables in the diet.

Duration of administration
No restrictions known.

Restrictions on use
A practitioner should be consulted if there is any doubt as to the nature of the problem, if symptoms persist unchanged for more than one week, or if there is a fever or blood in the urine.

Contra-indications
None known.

Pregnancy and nursing
It should not be used during pregnancy and breastfeeding. Nephrosolid may be taken instead for cystitis in pregnancy.

Adverse reactions
None known.

Ingredients

Arctostaphylos uva-ursi	25 per cent
Echinacea purpurea	25 per cent
Achillea millefolium	10 per cent
Hypericum perforatum	10 per cent
Avena sativa	10 per cent
Melissa officinalis	6 per cent
Rhus aromatica	5 per cent
Monarda didyma	5 per cent
Populus tremula	4 per cent

Application
Cystitis; urinary tract infections; bedwetting.

Cystitis is the term given to inflammation of the bladder. It arises most commonly as a result of bacterial infection but may also be caused by fungal infections and dietary factors. Infections of the bladder may track upwards towards the ureters and kidneys, causing more generalised infections of the urinary tract.

Symptoms of cystitis include urinary frequency, burning or scalding on passing urine, pain in the groin and a desire to pass water even though the bladder is empty.

Uva-ursi works as a urinary antiseptic. Its action is of benefit in cystitis caused by bacteria or fungi.

Rhus aromatica is a herb which is specific for bedwetting. Its action is aided by the astringent effect of *uva-ursi*, as well as the ability for *Hypericum perforatum* to 'tone up' the nervous system.

VALERIANA

Description
A fresh herbal extract of *Valeriana officinalis*, a herb which is widely used across Europe as a natural sedative for excitability and sleep disturbances.

Mode of action
Anxiolytic; tranquilliser; muscle relaxant.

The tranquillising action of *Valeriana officinalis* (valerian) has been attributed to a number of components.

A group of components known as valepotriates have an antispasmodic action and these, together with some of their breakdown products (baldrinals), have a depressant action on the central nervous system (CNS).

The volatile oil contains valerenone and valerenic acid. Valerenic acid inhibits the breakdown of the CNS neurotransmitter gamma-amino-butyric acid increasing its level in the brain with a consequent decrease in CNS activity. This reduction in nervous system activity helps people who find it hard to 'switch off', enhancing the natural body processes of slipping into sleep, reducing the frequency of waking and improving the quality of sleep. The herb has also been shown to improve the physical symptoms associated with anxiety and tension.

The advantage of using valerian to aid sleep is that it is unlikely to cause the drowsy hangover effect which may be experienced in the morning with pharmaceutical sedative preparations.

Valerenone present in the oil fraction has been shown to have a direct action on smooth muscle. This, together with the spasmolytic effects of the valepotriates, relaxes over-contracted muscles, which can be responsible for symptoms such as neck and shoulder tension, colic, period pain and high blood pressure, brought about through stress and anxiety. Nervous tension can often be a contributory factor to raised blood pressure and in these cases valerian is a useful herb which can be taken alongside pharmaceutical medication.

Dosage information
ADULTS: 10 drops in a little water three times a day. Before bedtime take 30 drops in a little water.

CHILDREN: If there are sleep problems associated with hyperactivity, then Dormeasan should be given.

Duration of administration
There are no restrictions on the long-term use of Valerian.

Restrictions on use
None known.

Contra-indications
The CNS depressant activity of Valerian may potentiate the effects of existing sedative therapy. Valerian does not potentiate the sedative effects of alcohol.

Pregnancy and nursing
Not recommended without medical supervision.

Adverse reactions
None known.

Ingredients
Valeriana officinalis 100 per cent
(Alcohol content: approximately 66 per cent)

Application
Anxiety/nervous tension; sleep disturbances associated with nervous overactivity; muscle tension and spasm.

Stress is a feature of modern living. While everyone needs some degree of stress, the level at which we are able to cope varies from one individual to another. If the level of stress exceeds the ability to cope, physical and behavioural symptoms associated with anxiety and tension may develop. These symptoms include problems sleeping, feelings of panic, poor concentration, tremors, palpitations and sweating.

Valerian has been known as herbal 'diazepam', beneficial in alleviating symptoms associated with anxiety and nervous tension. It has a calming action on the nervous system without the side effects of addiction, drowsiness, poor co-ordination and interaction with alcohol, which can be associated with conventional medicines.

❦ VALERIAN–HOPS COMPLEX ❦

Description
Valerian–Hops Complex, formerly known as Dormeasan, combines the sedative properties of valerian (*Valeriana officinalis*) and hops (*Humulus lupulus*) in a remedy to help with sleep disorders.

Valerian is found very commonly in all parts of Europe. It is the root which is used medicinally and the action of this plant has been exploited in European herbal medicines for many centuries.

Hop is a climbing plant which can be found in swamps and hedges. The seed-like fruit is an important ingredient in beer, so the plant is now cultivated commercially. Hop has a long history of use in phytotherapy; it was listed in the *US Pharmacopeia* from 1831 to 1916 as a sedative.

Mode of action
Sedative; relaxant.

Hop is a very useful agent for restlessness, overexcitability, anxiety, tension and sleep problems. It contains umulones and lupulones, which are metabolised in the body to a compound known as 2-methyl-3-buten-2-ol, which exerts a sedative effect on the central nervous system (CNS). It is also an antispasmodic bitter, enhancing digestion and easing intestinal tension.

Valerian is an herbal tranquilliser with a well-established use in those with nervous excitement and disturbed sleep patterns. It improves the ability to fall asleep and sleep quality. The relaxing properties are due to the valepotriates and volatile oils present (especially valerenal and valerenic acid). Valerenic acid inhibits the breakdown of the neurotransmitter GABA (gamma-amino-butyric acid), increasing its concentration. This then leads to a decrease in CNS activity and sedation.

Dosage information
ADULTS: 20–30 drops in a little water half an hour before bedtime.
CHILDREN: Half adult amount.
INFANTS: Up to five drops before bedtime.

This product can safely be used in hyperactive children and teething babies (put drops in fruit juice if needed).

Duration of administration
No restrictions to long-term usage known.

Restrictions on use
None known.

Contra-indications
None known.

This preparation should not be used to replace prescribed tranquillisers without medical supervision. It may, however, be used as an adjunct to such treatment. It may also be used for both acute and chronic disorders.

Pregnancy and nursing
To be avoided unless taken under the supervision of a practitioner.

Adverse reactions
None known.

Ingredients

Valeriana officinalis	50 per cent
Humulus lupulus	50 per cent

(Alcohol content: approximately 52 per cent)

Application
Mild insomnia; nervous tension (restlessness, excitability); hyperactive children; teething babies.

Difficulty getting off to sleep and disturbed sleep patterns are often associated with the pace of life today. Many herbs with sedative and hypnotic properties can help resolve this problem without the addictive and 'hangover' effects associated with many modern drugs. Both valerian and hops serve this purpose admirably, being the standard herbs used by many phytotherapists.

The gentle action of these herbs on the nervous system makes them suitable for use in children who are overactive, being restless and irritable as a result of teething or colic.

❧ VIOLA ❧

Description
This is a fresh extract of *Viola tricolor* (wild pansy), which has a traditional use as an 'alterative' or a 'depurative'. As these terms

suggest, *Viola tricolor* has a non-specific cleansing action which may be beneficial in many skin conditions.

The herb Viola is very commonly found in Europe. Two varieties may be found in the wild but the cultivated species are much more commonly encountered in our gardens.

Mode of action
Dermatrophic (skin nourishing properties); anti-inflammatory; diuretic.

Viola tricolor contains saponins. These soap-like molecules are able to soothe inflamed areas and, in part, are responsible for the soothing effect of the herb when applied externally.

The saponin component also makes Viola an 'eliminative' remedy. Blood flow to the kidneys is enhanced, with the elimination of toxins.

Viola tricolor also contains high levels of flavonoids, which have the ability to stabilise the capillary membranes. This is important in inflammatory conditions, especially those of the skin.

It has a gentle action, making it suitable for internal or external use in both children and adults.

Dosage information
ADULTS: 15–20 drops in water twice a day taken internally.
CHILDREN: Half adult amount.
INFANTS: Three to five drops in a little water up to three times a day.
EXTERNALLY: Use the Viola skin care range.

Duration of administration
No restrictions to long-term usage known.

Restrictions on use
None known.

Contra-indications
None known.

Pregnancy and nursing
Viola tricolor is not recommended during pregnancy without medical supervision.

Adverse reactions
None known.

Ingredients

Viola tricolor   100 per cent
(Alcohol content: approximately 43 per cent)

Application

Non-specific skin rashes; eczema; cradle cap.

Eczema is a common, itchy, inflammatory skin condition which is manifested in a number of different ways. Most often encountered are:

◆ Contact eczema, which is triggered by external irritants such as detergents, skin products and jewellery.

◆ Atopic eczema, which may be hereditary and usually appears in the elbow and knee flexures, ankles or face. Dietary factors are also involved.

Depuratives are blood cleansers which encourage removal of waste products. They possess a purifying action which can relieve symptoms associated with eczematous skin conditions. *Viola tricolor* has been used for many years to treat eczema. There has been a collection of reports on the benefits of this herb in both adults and infants. Weiss reports that paediatricians have seen excellent results in infants.

❧ YARROW COMPLEX ❧

Description

Yarrow Complex was previously known as Gastrosan. It is a herbal 'digestive tonic' containing a combination of bitter and aromatic herbs. The preparation has a wide spectrum of action and may be used in many of the common gastrointestinal complaints to stimulate digestion.

Bitter herbs have been known to phytotherapists for many years. These herbs are simply defined as those which are bitter to taste and many herbs have bitter properties. To phytotherapists, however, bitter herbs are those which can cause a clinically useful increase in gastric juice secretion.

Mode of action

Bitter tonic; digestive stimulant; carminative; antispasmodic; anti-inflammatory; stimulates secretion of bile.

All the herbs present in Yarrow Complex have bitter properties.

Gentian (*Gentiana lutea*), centaury (*Centaurium umbellatum*) and blessed thistle (*Carduus benedictus*) have the most prominent action. Dandelion (*Taraxacum officinale*) is a stomach bitter; it also acts as a liver tonic, enhancing liver function and bile production. Yarrow (*Achillea millefolium*), lemon balm (*Melissa officinalis*) and angelica (*Angelica archangelica*) contain volatile oils and flavonoids. These have an antispasmodic and anti-inflammatory action in the digestive system, easing colic and reducing flatulence.

Dosage information
ADULTS: 20–30 drops in a little water three times a day.
CHILDREN: Half adult amount.

Individual differences to the response to bitter herbs may sometimes require an adjustment to the recommended dosage.

Ideally, Yarrow Complex should be taken 15 minutes before meals in a little water. It should be sipped and held in the mouth before swallowing to encourage its bitter action.

Duration of administration
Yarrow Complex is suitable for long-term use. However, a break is often suggested, as continuous use may reduce its bitter action.

Restrictions on use
None. Certain individuals may be allergic to Achillea. Sunbathing should be avoided while taking Yarrow Complex, as a photosensitive reaction may occur with this herb.

Pregnancy and nursing
It should not be taken during pregnancy.

Adverse reactions
None known.

Ingredients
Achillea millefolium	29.5 per cent
Taraxacum officinales	22.0 per cent
Melissa officinalis	18.5 per cent
Gentiana Lutea	17.0 per cent
Carduus benedictus	7.0 per cent
Angelica archangelica	3.0 per cent
Centaurium umbellatum	3.0 per cent

(Alcohol content: approximately 60 per cent)

Application

General indigestion; poor or weak digestion; lack of appetite/anorexia; colic, wind and bloating; food allergies.

One of the key features of this remedy is its 'bitter action'. A bitter substance stimulates certain taste buds in the mouth, which increases the flow of saliva. More importantly, it increases the production of digestive enzymes through a reflex action mediated via the autonomic nervous system. This action improves the function of the organs responsible for the first part of the digestive process, enabling the body to utilise foods and absorb minerals more effectively.

Bitters are also useful in children with a poor appetite, and the elderly where, in the absence of an underlying physiological disturbance, dwindling saliva and enzyme activity may be the cause of anorexia.

In the use of bitter herbs, the bitter taste is essential to its therapeutic action and bitters in tablet or capsule form are ineffective.

JAN DE VRIES

I gained a lot of knowledge and experience working with Dr Vogel and started to develop my own remedies. I have found the following complexes particularly useful.

❧ ALOE VERA COMPLEX ❧

Description
Aloe Vera Complex is prepared from a number of freshly harvested herbs, formulated to help improve the distressing symptoms associated with psoriasis.

Mode of action
Nutritive; digestive stimulant; increases bile secretion; anti-inflammatory; nervous system relaxant.

It has been suggested that in psoriasis the incomplete digestion of protein produces toxic compounds which then promote abnormal cell proliferation in the skin. Impaired liver function, high alcohol and animal fat consumption are factors which have been implicated. Enhancing digestive function and especially the breakdown of protein encourages a better metabolism which helps to redress the imbalance.

The whole leaf of aloe vera (*Aloe barbadensis*) contains anthraquinone glycosides, resins and polysaccharides. Anthraquinones have a stimulating laxative action, which improves bowel function, eliminates wastes and relieves constipation, which is often a factor in psoriasis. The polysaccharides have an application in many skin conditions, possessing anti-inflammatory and immunomodulating activity. The gel itself contains 18 amino acids and vitamins.

German chamomile (*Matricaria recutita*) and Roman chamomile (*Anthemis nobilis*) possess similar pharmacological activities. The azulenes of the volatile oil possess anti-inflammatory activity. Bisabolol compounds and flavonoids in German chamomile are also anti-inflammatory.

The action of cardamon (*Elettaria cardamomum*) is mediated through its volatile oil component, which improves digestive function through its antispasmodic, carminative and stimulant action.

Enhancing liver function is considered by phytotherapists to be very important in psoriasis, as the liver is the main organ of metabolism. Silymarin, the main active constituent of milk thistle (*Silybum marianum*) improves liver function, inhibits inflammation and reduces excessive cellular proliferation.

Dosage information

ADULTS: 15–20 drops in water twice a day. For maintenance, 20 drops in water once a day.
CHILDREN: Not to be taken unless under medical supervision.

Duration of administration
No restrictions known.

Restrictions on use
None known.

Contra-indications
None known.

Pregnancy and nursing
It should not be taken during pregnancy.

Adverse reactions
None known.

Ingredients

Aloe barbadensis	30 per cent
Matricaria recutita	20 per cent
Anthemis nobilis	20 per cent
Elettaria cardamomum	20 per cent
Silybum marianum	10 per cent

(Alcohol content: approximately 65 per cent)

Application
Psoriasis.

Psoriasis is a common skin disorder which may be associated with serious emotional and psychological implications. It occurs equally in both sexes, at any age, but has a peak incidence in the 20–35 age group. The precise cause of psoriasis is unknown, although the family history is observed to be relevant. Emotional disturbances, hormonal factors, skin trauma, streptococcal infections and certain drugs may precipitate attacks. The commonest form of psoriasis, seen as red raised patches covered with silvery scales, occurs because the cells of the epidermis (the outermost layer of skin) divide ten times faster than normal. Common sites affected include the scalp, elbows, knees and lower back. In about 25 per cent of people the nails are affected with signs of 'pitting'. Arthritis can also be associated with psoriasis.

In phytotherapy, skin disease is seen as an external manifestation of an internal imbalance. An inadequate breakdown and elimination of toxins by the liver, digestive tract and kidneys will reflect in the health of the skin.

🦋 BLACK COHOSH 🦋

Description
A fresh herbal extract of the root of the black cohosh (*Cimicifuga racemosa*). It is a member of the buttercup family, originally used by native Americans for its 'normalising' and relaxant effects on the female reproductive system. In modern phytotherapy, black cohosh is used particularly for painful periods and problems associated with the menopause.

Mode of action
Oestrogen-like action; reduction in lutenising hormone release from the pituitary gland.

Black cohosh contains several important constituents – Triterpene glycosides (actein, cimicifugoside), isoflavones (formononetin) and salicylic acid. Triterpene glycosides such as cimicifugoside have an effect on the hypothalamus–pituitary system, reducing the concentration of lutenising hormone (LH). This in turn decreases progesterone production from the ovaries. Formononetin has been found to act on oestrogen receptors. However, it does not reduce serum LH levels. Clinical trials have shown that black cohosh is useful for hot flushes and the emotional problems associated with menopause which would normally benefit from hormone replacement therapy.

The mode of action of black cohosh in the treatment of menstrual difficulties is not clear. It seems to act both directly on the tissues of the reproductive system and indirectly through the nervous system. Clinical evidence has shown hypotensive, vasodilatory and anti-inflammatory activity. Actein, one of the triterpene glycosides, causes peripheral vasodilation and an increase in peripheral blood flow.

Black cohosh contains a natural source of salicylic acid,

which has an anti-inflammatory and mild analgesic action in painful inflammatory conditions.

Dosage information
ADULTS: 15–20 drops in water twice a day. For maintenance, 20 drops in water taken once a day.
CHILDREN: Not to be taken unless under medical supervision.

Duration of administration
A break is suggested after six months' continual use.

Restrictions on use
None known.

Contra-indications
None known.

Pregnancy and nursing
It should not be taken during pregnancy.

Adverse reactions
Gastrointestinal disturbances are occasionally experienced. Should not be taken by those allergic to aspirin.

Ingredients
Cimicifuga racemosa 100 per cent
(Alcohol content: approximately 65 per cent)

Application
Dysmenorrhoea; menopausal symptoms; premenstrual tension.

Two types of dysmenorrhoea (painful periods) can affect women. Primary (spasmodic) dysmenorrhoea is experienced in younger women. It is caused by the unco-ordinated uterine contractions which occur at the start of a period. This produces a colicky pain in the lower abdomen, back and legs, which can last for up to 48 hours.

Secondary (congestive) dysmenorrhoea occurs more often in older women. It may be caused by factors such as pelvic inflammatory disease, pelvic congestion, endometriosis, pelvic adhesions or fibroids. The pain starts as a dull ache in the lower abdomen or lower back.

Black cohosh is particularly effective at easing uterine cramps. It alters the oestrogen/progesterone balance in favour of oestrogen. This makes it useful for menopausal and menstrual problems associated with depression, where a dominance of progesterone is believed to play a part.

♥ FEVERFEW ♥

Description
This is the fresh herbal extract of feverfew (*Tanacetum parthenium*). The herb has been found to be beneficial in the treatment and prevention of migraine headaches.

Feverfew has daisy-like flowers, which is a characteristic of the *Compositae* family to which it belongs. The herb contains sesquiterpene lactones, volatile oils, pyrethrin flavonoids and tannins.

Mode of action
Inhibits serotonin release from platelets; inhibits platelet aggregation; reduces blood vessel constriction; inhibits formation and release of inflammatory substances.

Migraine is the result of an inflammatory phenomenon which occurs in the blood vessels surrounding the brain. Platelets of migraine sufferers have been demonstrated to aggregate (clump) more readily than those of others. This occurs both spontaneously and when exposed to serotonin and catecholamines such as adrenaline. If the blood levels of catecholamines rise, serotonin, which is a potent vasoconstrictor, is released. This causes platelet aggregation and vasospasm (spasm of blood vessels) which then leads to an interruption of blood flow to the brain. This is then followed by a 'rebound' vasodilation (widening of the blood vessels) and then the release of pain-inducing substances. This sequence of events leads to the characteristic symptoms associated with a migraine headache.

Sesquiterpene lactones, particularly parthenolide, are thought to be the main active constituents of feverfew. They inhibit platelet aggregation and the secretion of serotonin, which can trigger the vasoconstriction leading to a migraine.

Dosage information
ADULTS: 15–20 drops in water twice a day. For maintenance, 20 drops in water taken once a day.

ACUTE CONDITIONS: Eight drops every two hours for five doses, then 15–20 drops in water once a day.

CHILDREN: Not to be used unless under medical supervision.

Duration of administration

No restrictions known. Longer-term use is recommended for the treatment and prevention of migraine headaches.

Restrictions on use

None known.

Contra-indications

Those with a known hypersensitivity to other members of the *Compositae* family, such as chamomile or yarrow, may also be allergic to Feverfew. Feverfew should not be used by individuals who develop a rash on contact with the plant.

Pregnancy and nursing

Feverfew is contra-indicated during pregnancy because of its stimulant action on the womb.

Adverse reactions

Mouth ulcers, swollen lips and gastrointestinal upset may occur in rare cases. The time of onset of side effects is variable, with symptoms being apparent within the first week of treatment or appearing gradually over the first two months.

Ingredients

Tanacetum parthenium 100 per cent
(Alcohol content: approximately 65 per cent)

Application

Migraine headaches.

Migraine is a surprisingly common disorder, affecting 15–20 per cent of men and 25–30 per cent of women. It is characterised by recurrent attacks of headaches which are variable in intensity, frequency and duration. Attacks are commonly unilateral (on one side of the head) and associated with nausea, vomiting and loss of appetite. Certain factors have been identified which may contribute to migraine headaches. In women they are often related to the menstrual cycle, starting around puberty and continuing until the menopause. The cause of migraines has been attributed to an abnormal sensitivity of the blood vessels in the cerebral circulation. This results in an interference of blood flow in the cerebral cortex of the brain.

Emotional and psychological factors such as stress, tension, anxiety, fatigue or pain, are often trigger factors. Foods which contain vasoactive amines, such as chocolate, cheese and dairy products, citrus fruit, alcohol (especially red wine), red meats, tea, coffee and shellfish, are common triggers.

❦ GINGER ❦

Description
This is the fresh extract of ginger rhizome (*Zingiber officinalis*). This herb is used traditionally to help alleviate motion sickness and for reducing morning sickness during pregnancy.

Ginger belongs to the family *Zingiberaceae*. It is native to south-east Asia, where it is used extensively in cooking (not only for its flavour but as a preservative), but is cultivated in many other tropical countries. Ginger plays an important role in the traditional medicine of the West Indies, India and China.

Mode of action
Anti-emetic (antinausea); carminative; antispasmodic; circulatory stimulant; anti-inflammatory; diaphoretic.

The main active constituents of ginger appear to be the oleo-resins, particularly gingerols and shogaols and a volatile oil. Gingerols and shogaols give ginger its characteristic taste and these components inhibit nausea and vomiting. As a digestive tonic, ginger improves the production and secretion of bile, aids fat breakdown and lowers blood cholesterol levels. It speeds up the digestive process, allowing quicker transport of substances through the digestive tract. This lessens the irritation to the intestinal wall, easing flatulence and intestinal spasms.

Ginger has also been shown to improve the circulation by inhibiting platelet aggregation.

In conditions associated with fever, such as colds and flu, ginger acts as a useful diaphoretic (promoting perspiration – which helps bring down a high temperature) and increasing the elimination of toxins through the skin.

Ginger may also be useful in inflammatory joint diseases. The gingerols have been shown to inhibit the formation of pro-inflammatory substances such as leukotrienes and the prostaglandins involved in the inflammatory process.

Dosage information
ADULTS: 15–20 drops in water twice a day. For maintenance, 20 drops in water taken once a day.

CHILDREN: Half the adult amount.
MOTION SICKNESS: Ginger works best when taken two days
before a journey and continued during the journey.

Duration of administration
No restrictions known.

Restrictions on use
None known.

Contra-indications
None known.

Pregnancy and nursing
Do not exceed dosage instructions during pregnancy.

Interactions
None known.

Adverse reactions
Some people may experience heartburn or may be sensitive to
the taste of ginger.

Ingredients
Zingiber officinalis 100 per cent
(Alcohol content: approximately 65 per cent)

Application
Motion sickness; nausea and vomiting associated with pregnancy; poor peripheral circulation.

Nausea and vomiting are common symptoms of early pregnancy, occurring in up to 80 per cent of women. The cause of these symptoms is unknown. One theory suggests a temporary impairment of liver function. As the liver is responsible for detoxifying hormones, the increased levels of these substances stimulate the emetic (nausea and vomiting) centre located in the brain.

Motion sickness is common in children and also affects some adults when travelling by road, sea or air. Symptoms include dizziness, disturbed vision, nausea, cold sweats and pallor. These are thought to be induced as a result of conflicting messages to the emetic centre from visual, gastrointestinal and vestibular (inner ear) sources. Ginger seems to be effective in reducing motion sickness. It acts on the gastrointestinal tract itself rather than on the vestibular apparatus.

❧ KAVA-KAVA ❧

Description
A fresh herbal tincture prepared from the root of kava-kava (*Piper methysticum*). This plant is a perennial shrub belonging to the pepper family and may be found in nearly all the Pacific islands.

The ceremonial drinking of kava-kava has taken place on these islands for centuries and is an important part of its culture. Traditionally, the herb is used to induce calm. Over-indulgence of the herb produces euphoria and intoxication, perhaps accounting for its long-standing reputation as an aphrodisiac.

Mode of action
Anxiolytic (anti-anxiety); sedative; muscle relaxant; analgesic; local anaesthetic action.

The major components of kava-kava root are the kava lactones (also known as kava pyrones), which are comprised mainly of kavain, dihydrokavain and methysticin.

The action of kava lactones in reducing anxiety differs from that of the benzodiazepines, tricyclic antidepressants and the herb *Valeriana officinalis*. It does not interact with GABA (gamma-amin-butyric acid) or benzodiazepine sites in the brain; instead, it seems to act on the amygdalar complex in the limbic system of the brain, possessing the ability to block sodium channels, which, in turn, decreases nerve conduction.

Recent clinical studies have demonstrated the important role of kava-kava as a safe, non-addictive anxiolytic with an efficacy comparable to that of benzodiazepines such as valium or oxazepam. It has a non-sedative action with the advantage of improving memory and reaction time (which the benzodiazepine drugs reduce). A single higher dose taken at bedtime acts as a sedative in cases of mild insomnia.

Studies have also demonstrated the analgesic properties of kava lactones. Dihydrokavain has been shown to be more powerful than aspirin and seems to work through a non-opiate pathway.

Relaxation of smooth and skeletal muscle is also attributable to the kava lactones. These actions make kava-kava useful in conditions associated with muscle spasms or tension with accompanying pain (e.g. tension headaches).

Kava-kava exerts a local anaesthetic action on mucous membranes. A mouthwash could therefore be used to advantage in painful oral conditions such as mouth ulcers.

Dosage information

ADULTS: 15–20 drops in water twice a day. For maintenance, 20 drops in water taken once a day.

INSOMNIA: 20–30 drops in water to be taken one hour before bedtime.

CHILDREN: Not recommended.

Duration of administration

Long-term use is not recommended. A one-week break is suggested after each four weeks' usage.

Restrictions on use

Those using prescribed tranquillisers or medication for epilepsy should seek medical advice before using kava-kava.

Contra-indications

Kava-kava should not be taken at the same time as alcohol. It may potentiate the action of barbiturates, antidepressants and sedatives.

Pregnancy and nursing

Not recommended unless on medical advice.

Adverse reactions

A numbing sensation in the mouth which subsides quickly may be experienced on taking the tincture. This phenomenon is minimised by diluting the tincture in water and drinking the solution quickly.

Ingredients

Piper methysticum 100 per cent
(Alcohol content: approximately 67 per cent)

Application

Anxiety; insomnia; muscle tension.

Anxiety is a normal response to stress. It results in the sensation of 'butterflies in the stomach', a sense of fear or panic, which is experienced on occasions such as exams, driving tests and visits to the dentist. While for some, anxiety heightens performance, excessive anxiety can impair function. Individual variations in the tolerance levels to stress means that some people thrive on tension, while others with a lower tolerance become overwhelmed. For this group, the anxiety experienced is out of proportion to the cause.

Kava-kava has a useful role in the management of anxiety, as it has a central calming action on the brain. It also exhibits muscle relaxant activity.

❦ PEPPERMINT COMPLEX ❦

Description
Peppermint Complex is a fresh herb tincture which can help improve the symptoms associated with irritable bowel syndrome (IBS). The combination of herbs present are known to improve digestive function.

Mode of action
Smooth muscle relaxant (antispasmodic); digestive stimulant; carminative; stimulates bile secretion; bitter tonic; astringent; anti-inflammatory.

Peppermint (*Mentha piperita*) reduces nausea, colic, bloating and wind. It soothes an irritated bowel and relaxes smooth muscles in the colon. In total, this helps to reduce diarrhoea and relieve colonic spasm. These actions are largely due to the presence of volatile oils (especially menthol) which are carminatives and potent spasmolytics. This encourages smooth muscle relaxation, reducing sphincter tone and increasing bowel peristalsis.

Flavonoids present in peppermint also contribute to the spasmolytic activity and phenolic acids improve bile flow.

Fennel (*Foeniculum vulgare*) and angelica (*Angelica archangelica*) share a complementary carminative and antispasmodic action due to the presence of volatile oils and flavonoids.

Centaury (*Centaurium umbellatum*) has a bitter action which strengthens gastric function. It stimulates digestive secretion, hastening the breakdown of food. This in turn reduces nausea, heartburn and indigestion.

Tormentil (*Potentilla tormentilla*) contains tannins which act as a gentle tonic astringent for the symptoms associated with IBS.

Liquorice (*Glycyrrhiza glabra*) has an anti-inflammatory, demulcent action, which is useful for dyspepsia and inflammatory conditions of the digestive system.

Dosage information
ADULTS: 15–20 drops in water twice a day. For maintenance, 20 drops in water taken once a day.
CHILDREN: Not to be taken unless under medical supervision.

Duration of administration
No restrictions known.

Restrictions on use
None known.

Contra-indications
As this product contains liquorice, medical advice should be sought if individuals are taking medication for hypertension or diabetes. Note, however, that this component only makes up 5 per cent of the product.

Pregnancy and nursing
It should not be taken during pregnancy.

Adverse reactions
Angelica contains furanocoumarins, which may cause photosensitisation.

Ingredients
Mentha piperita	30 per cent
Centaurium umbellatum	25 per cent
Potentilla tormentilla	25 per cent
Foeniculum vulgare	10 per cent
Glycyrrhiza glabra	5 per cent
Angelica archangelica radix	5 per cent

(Alcohol content: approximately 63 per cent)

Application
Irritable bowel syndrome.

IBS is the commonly encountered functional disorder of the gastrointestinal tract. Female sufferers outnumber males by about two to one. The problem is characterised by recurrent episodes of abdominal discomfort, pain and altered bowel habit. Constipation or diarrhoea may be the major presenting feature. The pain experienced may be colicky or a continual dull ache often in the lower abdomen. Frequently, the pain is relieved through defecation or passing wind. Symptoms may be aggravated by emotional stress, anxiety or depressive disorders.

Those who suffer from IBS often have high stress levels and symptoms often occur in relation to a stressful life event. In some, dietary factors (e.g. caffeine) may trigger symptoms. Research has suggested that IBS may be associated with a generalised hypersensitivity of the smooth muscle in the digestive tract. This may explain how herbs such as peppermint, which reduces spasm in the colon, can reduce the pain associated with IBS.

I have greatly admired Dr Edward Bach who, in 1936, discovered the signatures and characteristics of certain flowers and devised 38 healing remedies, based on the properties of these flowers (see page 103). When I came to Britain I found that little was known of these remedies. Television presenter Gloria Hunniford and I started to promote them, and they soon became household friends.

Although I still use Bach remedies, I developed a few new remedies which I felt were needed to treat the emotional problems of everyday life in the twentieth and twenty-first centuries.

My combination flower essences are excellent on their own or accompanying another remedy.

❦ BOWEL ESSENCE ❦

Use
Can be used to avoid or lessen bouts of irritable bowel syndrome, Crohn's disease, and other bowel problems triggered by emotional stress and worry.

Ingredients
TORMENTIL: Beneficial for intestinal problems, especially where diarrhoea and constipation alternate. Alleviates the 'grippy' type of pain in the intestines.

CENTAURY: Gives inner strength and increases self-esteem. Alleviates nervous tension in the stomach area.

KAPOK BUSH: Promotes determination, resilience and 'grit'. (Origin: Australian bush.)

PEPPERMINT: Reduces nervousness and cramps in the stomach area. Helps to promote concentration, mental clarity, overcoming sluggishness and lethargy.

CHAMOMILE: Calms distraught emotions, soothing and relaxing the nerves. Decreases inner tension and disharmony. Helps to release tension and calms the mind and body.

YARROW: For those who are oversensitive and vulnerable. Brings about strength in emergency situations, helping to deal with problems. Harmonises the emotions, restores energy levels when involved in sudden shocks.

DANDELION: Reduces emotional tension held in the stomach muscles. Helps to soothe emotional issues. On a physical level, it removes excess water and promotes the formation of bile. Harmonises the physical and emotional aspects of the body.

🦋 CHILD ESSENCE 🦋

Use
Calming and soothing for nervous, hyperactive children. Good for bedwetting and helps poor sleepers. Assists in balancing children with dyslexia and concentration problems. Helps children adjust to new situations, e.g. a new school.

Ingredients
IMPATIENS: Brings about patience, reduces anger, irritability and restlessness. Promotes tolerance to those around us.

WILD OAT: Ideal as a nerve tonic, especially in bedwetting children. For children who are constantly seeking and who have a restless manner.

BLACK-EYED SUSAN: Reduces anger. For children who are constantly 'on the go', continually expending energy. (Origin: Australian bush and Californian deserts.)

MARIPOSA LILY: Ideal essence for children. Promotes the bonding with parents, especially mothers. Brings about a sense of nurturing, warmth, being part of a family group and belonging. Promotes a sense of security, confidence, trust and calm. (Origin: California deserts.)

CHAMOMILE: Calms distraught emotions, soothing and relaxing

the nerves. Decreases inner tension and disharmony. Helps to release tension and calms the mind and body.

❧ CONCENTRATION ESSENCE ❧

Use
Helps the mind to focus. Helpful when preparing for exams, important interviews, etc. Also good for dyslexia, dyspraxia and stutters, as it balances the left and right sides of the brain.

Ingredients
GINKGO BILOBA: Balances the left and right sides of the brain. Brings about mental clarity. Can be taken by people with dyslexia and stuttering.

SIBERIAN GINSENG: Stimulates the central nervous system and the endocrine system. Co-ordinates and stimulates, bringing the mind, body and spirit into harmony. This essence can be seen as the catalyst around which all others are drawn. Blends both male and female energies. Protects against stress.

COSMOS: Helps those who are introverted, shy and who have difficulty in expressing themselves. Will promote composure. It concentrates the mind before speaking, increasing linguistic ability. (Origin: America.)

MADIA: Brings the individual mental focus, concentration, attention to detail and promotes an ability to follow through with a project. Good for those who are easily distracted. This essence activates the creative power of an individual. (Origin: Europe and America.)

ROSEMARY: This essence brings clarity to a person's state of mind. Especially good for those who write much detail. Brings about a state of inner peace.

❧ EMERGENCY ESSENCE ❧

Use
Supportive in any stressful situation. Easy to use, works fast. Keep it with you – you never know when you might need it!

Ingredients
CHAMOMILE: Calms distraught emotions, soothing and relaxing the nerves. Decreases inner tension and disharmony.

Helps to release tension and calms the mind and body.

LAVENDER: Balances the emotions; good for those who are highly strung and tense. Soothes frayed nerves from overstimulation.

RED CLOVER: Helpful during emotionally charged family situations. Acts as a balancer, instilling calmness and clarity.

PURPLE CONEFLOWER: Overcomes fear in emergency situations and severe trauma. Restores balance when in shock and in traumatic situations. Brings a sense of security when feeling vulnerable.

SELF-HEAL: Eases self-doubt and confusion. General enhancer of well-being, promoting self-confidence and self-acceptance. Provides inner motivation to be well. Counteracts physical, psychological and emotional stress.

YARROW: For those who are oversensitive and vulnerable. Brings about strength in emergency situations, helping to deal with problems. Harmonises the emotions, restores energy levels when involved in sudden shocks.

❧ FEMALE ESSENCE ❧

Use
Unblocks the hormonal channels and hence has a hormonal balancing effect. Can be taken for PMT, menopausal problems and infertility with no known cause. Safe with other hormonal herbal remedies, the pill and HRT.

Ingredients
SHE-OAK: For hormonal imbalances in women. Helps with the inability to conceive for no physical reason, releasing the emotional blocks preventing conception. Increases self-confidence and esteem. (Origin: Australian bush.)

EVENING PRIMROSE: Used for depression due to rejection in childhood and a lack of emotional support during infancy. Helps to form relationships and increases emotional security.

LADY'S MANTLE: Harmonises the emotions with the reproductive organs to bring about a release in tension, especially during menstruation and menopause. It helps those women who wish to be in touch with the female power within.

LAVENDER: Balances the emotions; good for those who are highly strung and tense. Soothes frayed nerves from overstimulation.

MARIPOSA LILY: Promotes a sense of security, confidence, trust and calm. (Origin: Californian deserts.)

❧ MALE ESSENCE ❧

Use
Balances emotions and helps men to accept and express their true feelings. A stimulant for impotency. Boosts confidence, self-esteem and your sex life! General tonic to increase motivation.

Ingredients
AGRIMONY: Brings about self-worth and self-acceptance. Useful when emotions are covered up by false cheerfulness. Promotes acceptance of the true feelings which are often hidden from other people.

SEQUOIA: Gives strength to carry out daily tasks. Teaches responsibility, resourcefulness and steadfastness. (Origin: Californian deserts.)

STICKY MONKEY FLOWER: Dispenses with fear and confusion about sexual intimacy. Balances emotions about sexuality. Helps to remove emotional and mental blocks brought about by past experiences. (Origin: Californian deserts.)

FLANNEL FLOWER: For men who shy away from physical contact, fear of intimacy and for those who have a lack of sensitivity related to past trauma or hurt. It helps to increase trust and sensitivity. (Origin: Australian bush.)

SUNFLOWER: For low self-esteem and lack of confidence. Promotes leadership qualities. Balances and tempers the male ego from being too overbearing. (Origin: Mexico.)

DANDELION: Helps to soothe emotional issues. Harmonises the physical and emotional aspects of the body.

DAMIANA: Used as a stimulant for impotency and as an essence, helps to remove emotional and psychological barriers surrounding it. (Origin: America and Mexico.)

❦ VITALITY ESSENCE ❦

Use
Brilliant for hangovers (we're told). Increases energy levels and enthusiasm. Good for long drives, long meetings and that 3 p.m. energy slump. General tonic to increase motivation.

Ingredients
CAPERBERRY: Promotes energy, vitality and a zest for life.

ALOE VERA: Restores energy when feeling 'burnt out' or exhausted. Particularly good for workaholics.

OLIVE: Helpful for nervous tension. Restores peace of mind. Beneficial for those who have suffered from stress, trauma or illness for long periods of time. Promotes inner strength and gives the confidence to cope.

SIBERIAN GINSENG: Stimulates the central nervous system and the endocrine system. Co-ordinates and stimulates, bringing the mind, body and spirit into harmony. This essence can be seen as the catalyst around which all others are drawn. Blends both male and female energies. Protects against stress.

WILD ROSE: This is the essence of independence. It softens the emotions, overcomes apathy and a lack of motivation. Endows the individual with dynamic energy and enthusiasm.

ZINNIA: This essence promotes laughter and cheerfulness. It is useful for those who take themselves too seriously, with the tendency for working too hard and feeling overburdened by responsibilities. (Origin: America.)

BACH FLOWER REMEDIES

I will now follow with a brief description of Dr Bach's remedies and talk about two of my favourite and most-prescribed ones – Rescue Remedy and Rescue Cream – although I like all of them. These are very well provided by one of the oldest homoeopathic herbal companies in this country, for which I have great respect. As homoeopathic remedies in combination with herbal remedies, these combinations work very well.

The Bach Flower Remedies are 38 homoeopathically prepared plant- and flower-based remedies, each one devised to treat a specific emotion, helping to restore balance and overcome negative feelings which, if allowed to continue, can lead to physical illness. Dr Edward Bach, who originally created the flower remedies, believed a healthy mind ensures a healthy body.

Dr Bach also created an emergency combination which he called Rescue Remedy, one of the most-prescribed products. It contains five flower remedies: impatiens, star of Bethlehem, cherry plum, rock rose and clematis. It can be used to help someone to face a difficult situation – such as a family upset, the aftermath of an accident or other stressful event – in a better frame of mind, and can reduce fear or nervousness. It is an excellent remedy for general nervousness.

Rescue Cream is available as a multi-purpose skin salve for external applications.

ENZYMATIC THERAPY

When I worked in the USA, I discovered some remedies by a company called Enzymatic Therapy. I tried them out and found them to be very effective. Luckily I found a company in the UK which would import them for me. Long research has gone into these remedies and indeed they are used with great success. The following remedies are the ones that I work with the most.

🦋 VISION ESSENTIALS 🦋

This supplement contains vitamins essential for eye function, namely A, C and B2 (riboflavin), and bilberry extract.

Vitamins A and C are antioxidants, compounds that prevent tissue damage by free radicals, produced by metabolic processes and pollutants. Riboflavin helps regenerate antioxidants after they have neutralised free radicals. The bilberry extract is standardised for its content of anthocyanosides (flavonoid compounds that have natural antioxidant activity).

Ingredients
VITAMIN A (BETA-CAROTENE): An essential vitamin that is needed for growth and maintenance of the skin and proper function of the eye. This is also an important antioxidant.

VITAMIN C: Also an important antioxidant and essential for the growth and repair of tissues in all parts of the body.

RIBOFLAVIN (B2): This vitamin is essential for healthy eyes. Found in the pigment of the retina, it enables the eyes to adapt to light. Thus B2 deficiencies can manifest themselves as photophobia (excessive sensitivity to light that causes the eyes to water and become inflamed and bloodshot). Vision may become blurred and the eyes may easily become tired. Studies have shown that this vitamin may even prevent cataracts or delay their progress.

BILBERRY EXTRACT: Bilberries have, of course, been used as food and for their high nutritive value. Medicinally, they have been utilised in the treatment of scurvy and urinary complaints (including infection and stones). Renewed interest in the medicinal use of bilberry was first aroused when it was observed during the Second World War that British RAF pilots reported improved night-time visual acuity on bombing raids after consuming bilberries. Subsequent studies show that administration of bilberry extracts to healthy subjects results in improved night-time visual acuity, quicker adjustment to darkness, and faster restoration of visual acuity after exposure to glare.

Clinical Application

In Europe, bilberry extracts are now part of the conventional medical treatment for many eye disorders including cataracts and macular degeneration, as well as diabetic retinopathy and night blindness. This use is supported by positive results in controlled clinical trials.

The macula is the portion of retina in the eye that is responsible for fine vision; it is located at the centre of the retina. Degeneration of the macula is the leading cause of severe visual loss in the United States and Europe in persons aged 55 years or older. Presumably, the degeneration is a result of free radical damage similar to the type of damage that induces cataracts. The risk factors for macular degeneration include ageing, ateriosclerosis and hypertension.

Antioxidants and Free Radicals

Antioxidants are compounds that prevent free radical or oxidative damage. A free radical is a highly reactive molecule that can bind to and destroy cellular components. Free radical or oxidative damage initiates many degenerative processes in the body and is what makes us age.

Treatment

As with most things, prevention or treatment at an early stage is most effective. Since free radical damage and lack of blood and oxygen supply to the macula appear to be the primary factors in macular degeneration, individuals with macular degeneration should greatly increase intake of antioxidant nutrients. Although nutritional antioxidants (e.g. vitamins C and E, zinc and selenium) are important in the treatment of macular degeneration, standardised ginkgo biloba or bilberry extracts can offer even greater benefit.

Diet

Avoid rancid foods and other sources of free radicals. Increase consumption of legumes (high in sulphur-containing amino acids), yellow vegetables (carotenes), flavonoid-rich berries (bilberries, blackberries, cherries etc.) and vitamin E- and C-rich foods (fresh fruits and vegetables).

❦ GINKGO PHYTOSOME ❦

Ginkgo biloba has the ability to stimulate the circulation to the brain and periphery (hands and feet). It has become known as the memory tree since those using it reported improvements in short-term memory.

Herbs have been providing individuals with therapeutic benefit for centuries. Before there was aspirin, there was white willow; before there were antibiotics, there was goldenseal; and long before there was Tagamet® or Zantac®, there was liquorice extract.

The *ginkgo biloba* tree is the world's oldest living tree species. It can live as long as 1,000 years and may grow to a height of more than 100 feet with a diameter of three to four feet. Once common in North America and Europe, the ginkgo was almost destroyed during the Ice Age in all regions of the world except China, where it has long been cultivated as a sacred tree. In the late seventeenth century, a German physician and botanist became the first European to discover and catalogue the ginkgo tree. However, the medicinal use of ginkgo biloba can be traced back to the oldest Chinese *Materia Medica* (2800 BC). Traditional Chinese medicine prescribes ginkgo leaves for their ability to 'benefit the brain' and to relieve coughs and the symptoms of asthma.

In this product, the ginkgo is bound to a special nutrient called phosphatidylcholine. Phosphatidylcholine is a fat-soluble substance found throughout the body in cell membrane. It surrounds the water-soluble herbal molecule, resulting in an entirely new molecule, thus providing more benefit than the original herb alone. Phosphatidylcholine is also an emulsifier, allowing it to combine effectively materials that would normally not mix, such as fat-soluble and water-soluble molecules. The emulsifying action of the phosphatidylcholine is often used to increase the absorption of vitamins and drugs by the body.

The key benefits of the phytosome process are:

◆ Significantly improved absorption, three to seven times greater than non-phytosome products.
◆ Increased biological activity with the therapeutic properties of the herb lasting longer in the body – as much as twice as long in some cases.
◆ Enhanced and increased delivery of the health-promoting molecules with more of the herb getting into the body where it is needed most.

Clinical application

Some of the key medicinal uses of ginkgo biloba extract are: cerebral vascular insufficiency and impaired mental performance, Alzheimer's disease, cochlear (inner ear) deafness, senile macular degeneration and diabetic retinopathy, impotence, pre-menstrual syndrome, depression, allergies and asthma.

Dosage information

One to three capsules daily as an addition to the everyday diet. The colour of this capsule may vary from one batch to another, just as the colour of its natural ingredients may vary.

Each capsule contains Ginkgo Phytosome 80mg.

❧ SINUCOMP ❧

Description

An all-herbal formula containing:

Cowslip flowers (*Primula veris*)	36mg
Sour dock (*Rumex acetosa*)	36mg
Elderflowers (*Sambucus nigra*)	36mg
Verbena (*Verbena officinalis*)	36mg
Gentian root (*Gentiana lutea*)	12mg

This product has been developed in accordance with monograph standards set forth by the German Kommission. It contains no sugar, salt, yeast, wheat, gluten, corn, soy, dairy products, colouring, flavouring or preservatives.

Clinical application

This all-herbal formula is popular in Europe for supporting sinus cavities, especially the mucous membranes. For use on colds, allergies, and sinus inflammation.

Dosage information

One tablet three times a day.

Adverse reactions

No side effects have been reported with this remedy.

OSTEOPRIME

Description

Bone health is one of the main concerns reported by women, especially those who are passing through or are in the menopause. While diet is important in maintaining adequate calcium intake, and exercise is necessary to encourage bone strength and formation, some women may wish to supplement their diets with extra calcium. Extra calcium is important, but bones require more than one element for health and strength and large doses of calcium provide little help.

OsteoPrime was formulated for Enzymatic Therapy by Drs Jonathan Wright and Alan Gaby, who researched the nutritional requirements of bone and discovered that 22 nutrients were needed to keep this tissue healthy and strong. OsteoPrime contains all 22 of these nutrients.

Dosage information

Two tablets twice a day, during or after meals, as an addition to the daily diet.

Ingredients

Four tablets contain:

Vitamin D	200iu
Calcium (aspartate, citrate, succinate, fumarate, carbonate, lactate, malate)	600mg
Magnesium (aspartate, oxide)	250mg
Vitamin C (ascorbic acid)	100mg
Vitamin B6 (pyridoxine)	25mg
Niacinamide	20mg
Zinc (picolinate)	15mg
Manganese (aspartate)	15mg
Thiamine HCL (vitamin B1)	10mg
Riboflavin (vitamin B2)	10mg
Pantothenic acid (D-calcium pantothenate)	10mg
Copper (gluconate)	1.5 mg
Folic acid	400mcg
Vitamin K (phytonadione)	150mg
Chromium (aspartate)	100mg
Selenium (sodium selenite)	100mg
Molybdenum (sodium molybdate)	50mg
Vitamin B12 (cyanocobalamin)	10mg
Betaine HCL	20mg

Silicon (sodium metasilicate)	1mg
Boron (chelated)	750mg
Strontium (non-radioactive)	500mg

❧ OSTEOPOROSIS AND BONE HEALTH ❧

Osteoporosis literally means 'porous bone'. Normally there is a decline in bone mass after the age of 40 in both sexes (about 2 per cent loss per year), but women are at a much greater risk of osteoporosis because of lower bone density prior to the age of 40. The most common form of osteoporosis is post-menstrual osteoporosis – approximately one in four post-menopausal women have osteoporosis. Although the entire skeleton may be involved in post-menopausal osteoporosis, bone loss is usually greatest in the spine, hips and ribs. Since these bones bear a great deal of weight, they are susceptible to pain, deformity or fracture.

Major risk factors for osteoporosis in women
◆ Family history of osteoporosis
◆ Gastric or small bowel resection (removal)
◆ Heavy alcohol use
◆ Hyperparathyroidism
◆ Hyperthyroidism
◆ Inactivity
◆ Leanness
◆ Long-term glucocorticosteroid therapy
◆ Long-term use of anticonvulsants
◆ Low calcium intake
◆ Nulliparity (never having been pregnant)
◆ Post-menopause
◆ Premature menopause
◆ Short stature and small bones
◆ Smoking
◆ White or Asian race

Dietary and lifestyle recommendation
◆ Consume a diet which focuses on whole, unprocessed foods
◆ Eliminate the intake of alcohol, caffeine and sugar
◆ Do not drink soft drinks
◆ Get regular exercise – walking is very good
◆ Perform a relaxation exercise (deep breathing, meditation)
◆ Drink at least 48 fl oz of water a day

Supplementation

Bone is dynamic living tissue that is constantly being broken down and rebuilt, even in adults. Normal bone metabolism is dependent on an intricate interplay of many nutritional and hormonal factors, with the liver and kidneys having a regulatory effect as well.

Regular exercise and a healthy, calcium-rich diet helps build and maintain bones and may reduce the risk of osteoporosis, particularly for white and Asian women in their bone-forming years. By slowing the rate of bone loss, adequate calcium intake is also linked to a reduced risk of osteoporosis in post-menopausal women. However, daily intakes above 2,000mg are not likely to provide any additional benefit.

Bones need more than calcium. Vitamin D is necessary to utilise calcium and phosphorus properly. Magnesium activates enzymes that help form new calcium crystals. Vitamin K helps the body produce osteocalcin, the supporting structure on which the bone crystallises. Studies show that manganese, zinc, strontium, vitamin B6, vitamin C, silicon, copper and boron also help form the connective structures in the bone.

OsteoPrime

This comprehensive formula contains the correct ratio of calcium and other bone-building nutrients, all of which play an important role in the bone structure (as listed above). All these nutrients are conveniently provided in one tub (available in capsule or tablet form).

❧ OESTROGEN REPLACEMENT THERAPY ❧

What is menopause?

Simply put, menopause is when a woman stops menstruating. Menstruation may stop suddenly, there may be a decreased flow each month until a final cessation, or the interval between periods may be lengthened until complete cessation. Symptoms or side effects of menopause include one or more of the following: hot flushes, night sweats, insomnia, thinning of the vaginal lining and psychological effects such as depression, anxiety and forgetfulness.

Oestrogen therapy

The most popular treatment choice for menopause is the

prescription of synthetic oestrogen. While synthetic oestrogens will usually take care of menopausal hot flushes, they are not without side effects themselves.

The most popular synthetic oestrogen is Premarin, made from pregnant mare urine. Regarding Premarin, the Physician's Desk Reference (PDR) highlights: 'Oestrogens have been reported to increase the risk of endometrial carcinoma in post-menopausal women. Some studies have suggested a possible increased incidence of breast cancer in those women on oestrogen therapy taking higher doses for prolonged periods of time. A recent study has reported a 2.5-fold increase in the risk of surgically confirmed gallbladder disease in women receiving post-menopausal oestrogen.'

In addition, oestrogen therapy can cause numerous other side effects such as vaginal yeast infections, breast tenderness or enlargement, nausea, cramping, bloating, headache/migraine, changes in weight, depression and mood changes.

It is reported that of the women who do choose hormone replacement therapy, one-third stop within nine months and more than half within a year, due to side effects.

Most healthcare professionals prescribe oestrogen therapy to offset any risk of osteoporosis or heart disease. Unfortunately, studies indicate that as soon as oestrogen therapy is stopped, bone loss escalates, which means a woman would have to remain on the oestrogen forever. As noted above, long-term use of oestrogen is not recommended as it poses an increased risk of breast cancer. Oestrogen's cardiovascular benefits are debatable. Natural health experts agree that there are more appropriate ways to prevent heart disease than by taking prescription oestrogen.

Comprehensive care
A comprehensive approach to making a smooth menopausal transition should include:
◆ A healthy diet featuring lots of fresh fruits, vegetables, soy products and plenty of fresh water.
◆ Additional vitamin C (1,000 to 3,000mg daily).
◆ A comprehensive calcium/magnesium formulation to protect and maintain bone health, along with a comprehensive multivitamin mineral formula.
◆ Plenty of exercise, which will provide numerous health benefits.

With the proper natural support, menopause can be a very positive time. Listen to your body and take control of your situation. Look at this transition as a time of empowerment – a time to take care of yourself and look closely at what you need and want.

Phytoestrogens

Many plant extracts exhibit a tonic effect on the female glandular system. This tonic effect is thought to result from the action of phytoestrogens as well as from the plant extract's ability to improve blood flow to the female organs. The herbs work to nourish and tone the female glandular and organ system rather than exert a drug-like effect. This non-specific mode of action makes many herbs useful in a broad range of female conditions.

Phytoestrogens are components of many medicinal herbs historically used to treat conditions now treated with oestrogens. Phytoestrogen-containing herbs offer significant advantages over the use of oestrogens in the treatment of menopausal symptoms. While both synthetic and natural oestrogens may pose significant health risks, including increasing the risk of cancer, gallbladder disease and thromboembolic disease (strokes, heart attacks, etc.), phytoestrogens have not been associated with these side effects.

Phytoestrogens in herbs are capable of exerting oestrogenic effects, although the activity compared to oestrogen is only 2 per cent as strong as oestrogen, at the very most. However, because of this low activity, phytoestrogens exert a balancing action on oestrogen effects: if oestrogen levels are low, phytoestrogens enhance the oestrogen effects; if oestrogen levels are high, phytoestrogens reduce the oestrogen effects.

❧ PHYTOGEN ❧

Description

Phytogen is a unique combination of plant-derived oestrogens (phytoestrogens) and vitamin E. This product is a popular dietary supplement for women in mid-life.

Vitamin E has been associated with a healthy heart and circulatory system for a long time. Women need to take special care of this factor when approaching the menopause. The extracts obtained from the rice bran, known as gamma-oryzanol, have been studied for the beneficial effect ithey have on the various fats contained in the blood, while flaxseed oil helps support hormone function in combination with pumpkin seed and soya oil.

Dosage information
One to three capsules daily as an addition to the everyday diet.

Ingredients
Each capsule contains:

Vitamin E (D-alpha tocopherol)	150iu
Barlean's flaxseed oil	300mg
Gamma-oryzanol	100mg
Pumpkin seed oil (*Curcurbita pepo*)	50mg
Soy extract	20mg

❧ DAILY CHOICE ANTIOXIDANT ❧

Description
Every day we come into contact with a wide range of smoke, pollutants and other substances that place our bodies under constant attack. The end result is the production of highly reactive chemicals within the body known as free radicals. These can damage the health and well-being of every body tissue and must be neutralised by natural antioxidants produced by the body. In times of stress, general debility or exposure to pollution, the body may need a little assistance.

Daily Choice Antioxidant supplies a well-balanced and complete antioxidant protection and is derived from natural ingredients such as vitamins A, C and E, selenium, N-acetylcysteine (which helps to protect against all types of toxins, including cigarette smoke and alcohol), cabbage extract, garlic and green tea extract.

Dosage information
One capsule three times a day as an addition to the everyday diet.

Ingredients
Each capsule contains:

Non-toxic form of vitamin A (beta carotene)	10,000iu

Vitamin E (D-alpha tocopherol)	200iu
Vitamin C (ascorbic acid)	500mg
Zinc (picolinate)	15mg
Manganese (gluconate)	15mg
Riboflavin (vitamin B2)	6mg
Selenium (L-selenomethionine)	200mg
N-acetylcysteine	100mg
Cabbage extract (*Brassica oleracea*)	100mg
Garlic extract (deodorised)	100mg
Ginger root (*Zingiber officinalis*) extract (6.5:1)	100mg
Green tea (*Camellia sinensis*) extract	100mg
Klamath blue-green algae	100mg
Curcuma root (*Curcuma longa*) extract	50mg
Grape seed (PCO) extract	10mg

Contains no sugar, salt, yeast, wheat, corn, dairy products, colouring, flavouring or preservatives.

There is still no official endorsement for the use of antioxidant nutrients in the prevention of chronic disease, but there is compelling evidence to recommend them in addition to a balanced diet. This formula is one of the most complete currently available. I would suggest taking two capsules daily with food.

Antioxidants are compounds that prevent the free radical or oxidative damage that initiate many degenerative processes in the body, including ageing. Although the body's own generation of free radicals is important, the environment also contributes greatly to the free radical load. Environmental influences such as cigarette smoking, drugs, air pollutants, pesticides, anaesthetics, aromatic hydrocarbons, fried food, solvents, alcohol and ionising radiation can produce harmful effects and individuals exposed to these factors may need additional antioxidant support.

Daily Choice Antioxidant contains high concentrations of antioxidant nutrients in a base of unique herbal extracts and other natural compounds. Daily Choice Antioxidant is also rich in the vitamins and minerals that are essential for cellular health and detoxification functions. This helps to protect the cells from inside and out, in one complete formula.

❦ SUPER MILK THISTLE ❦

The liver is the most important organ in removing and eliminating toxic chemicals from the blood. Unfortunately, the liver was not designed to deal with the pollutants that have become a part of modern life. These pollutants can accumulate in the body and disrupt normal function. However, cleansing and detoxifying the body – by taking regular physical exercise and following a low-fat, high-complex-carbohydrate diet – can reverse this process.

There are a number of never-ending toxic substances that our bodies are subjected to each day. Environmental contamination due to industry is the primary source of the extremely toxic compounds known as heavy metals. These include lead, mercury, cadmium, arsenic, nickel and aluminium. Over a billion pounds of lead alone are dumped into our atmosphere each year by industrial sources and leaded petrol! Some of this lead is inhaled, some of it drifts onto our crop lands or into our water supplies. It is then ingested as we eat and drink. We are all exposed to an endless supply of inescapable substances that can stress the liver. Some of our customary habits can also expose us to other substances such as alcohol, food additives and some medicines.

The heavy metals tend to accumulate in the brain, kidneys and immune system and can disrupt normal function. Increased exposure to toxins of many kinds are linked to such physical problems as cancer, fatigue, headache, muscle pains, digestive disturbances and constipation. Other symptoms may occur, such as anaemia, pallor, dizziness and poor co-ordination. As well as physical problems, some may experience such mental problems as abnormal nerve reflexes, depression and mental confusion. Heavy metals can also be associated with criminal behaviour. However, 'getting the lead out' can reverse some of these problems.

Detoxifying

The first step to detoxifying is to adopt a healthy lifestyle by taking regular physical activity, which assists the digestive and detoxification process.

It is also important to have a low-fat, high-complex-carbohydrate diet. For detoxification it is helpful to be a bit more strict with the diet than usual. Eliminate all alcohol, sugar, saturated fats, drugs and any other substances that you suspect may be toxic to the liver. An important group of foods that are sources of water-soluble fibres are pears, apples, legumes and oat bran. Broccoli, cabbage and Brussels sprouts also play an important role. Herbs and spices like cinnamon, liquorice and garlic are helpful, as are beets, carrots, dandelion and artichokes. The very important foods are those high in sulphur: onions, garlic and legumes. In general, keep to fresh fruits and vegetables, whole grains, legumes, seeds and nuts.

Fasting is also a good option in a detoxifying programme. A form of fasting that is more prevalent than total abstinence is a juice fast. Typically, it will last three to five days. Three or four 8–12oz juice 'meals' are taken each day. Either the day before the fast, or at the last meal before the fast, it is recommended to have a meal of just fresh vegetables and fruits (ideally organic). During the fast, drink a lot of water, get good rest and keep warm. After the fast, reintroduce solid foods slowly, taking special care to chew the food thoroughly and not to overeat. Then, stay on a good, low-fat, high-complex-carbohydrate diet to let your body enjoy the benefits of the detoxification programme.

Enzymatic Therapy's Super Milk Thistle provides good support for detoxification.

Mode of action

MILK THISTLE EXTRACT: Stimulates the liver's production of antioxidants, helping prevent further damage. It also builds up the levels of glutathione, a small protein-based molecule that helps the body metabolise pesticides and other environmental toxins. It also stimulates protein synthesis, causing enhanced production of new liver cells to replace those that have been damaged.

DANDELION ROOT EXTRACT: Traditionally used as a liver 'tonic', it enhances the flow of bile, improving such conditions as liver congestion, bile duct inflammation, hepatitis, gallstones and jaundice. Dandelion affects the liver directly by causing an increase in bile production and flow to the gallbladder and it exerts a direct effect on the gallbladder, causing contraction and release of stored bile.

ARTICHOKE LEAVES EXTRACT: The artichoke has a long folk history in treating many liver diseases. The active ingredients in artichoke are caffeylquinic acids (like cynarin). These compounds have significant liver protecting and regenerating effects.

LIQUORICE EXTRACT: Studies show that it assists the liver in detoxification reactions, improves liver function and reduces blood levels of liver enzymes that signify liver damage.

❧ CANDIDA FORMULA AND ENZYDOPHILUS ❧

Yeast (also known as *Candida albicans*) is not a problem in itself. Generally, it lives harmlessly in the gastrointestinal tract, just a natural part of the human ecosystem. When this ecosystem is in the proper balance, the friendly bacteria in the body keep *candida* growth in check. However, this balance may be upset in people who have used antibiotics, birth-control pills, corticosteroids, anti-ulcer drugs or who consume a high sugar diet. This overgrowth is believed to cause a wide variety of symptoms in virtually every system of the body. The gastrointestinal, genito-urinary, endocrine, nervous and immune systems are the most susceptible. Many illnesses can be traced to *candida* overgrowth.

Individuals concerned about the balance of yeast in their body are recommended to restrict their intake of refined sugars, foods with a high mould content (alcohol, cheese, dried fruits, melons and peanuts), milk and milk products and carbohydrate vegetables (potatoes, corn and parsnips). A diet rich in vegetables (except those previously mentioned), low-fat protein, whole grains and fruits such as apples, blueberries, cherries, other berries and pears are recommended for *candida* sufferers. It is also important to support the digestive system, immune system and liver function.

Candida Formula

Because yeast balance is important for men, women and children, Enzymatic Therapy have developed an all-natural product called Candida Formula. This is a herbal complex to provide support for individuals on a yeast-restrictive programme.

Candida Formula provides high-quality extracts of oregano (aids the digestive system), thyme (mucus cleansing and antiseptic properties), peppermint oil (supports colon health, aids elimination of gas and helps promote flow of bile) and goldenseal root (antibiotic and anti-infective properties, helps increase blood flow to the spleen, therefore stimulating the immune system).

The volatile oils are the most important constituents of oregano and thyme. Scientists recognise the role these volatile oils play in the digestive process and other body functions. Oregano also contains alkaloids and thyme is a good source of flavonoids, saponins, triterpenes and tannins. Peppermint oil contains flavonoids, tocopherols, carotenoids, azulenes and rosmarinic acid. Goldenseal contains alkaloids such as hydrastine, berberine and canadine. Of these alkaloids, berberine has been the most widely studied. Research has shown a link between these natural compounds and the balance of *candida* in the body.

Enzydophilus

Probiotics, literally meaning 'for life', is a term used to signify the health-promoting effects of 'friendly bacteria'. There are at least 400 different species of microflora in the human gastrointestinal tract. The most important friendly bacteria are *Lactobacillus acidophilus* and *Bifidobacterium benfidum*. Both of these friendly bacteria can be found in the Enzymatic Therapy product Enzydophilus.

Enzydophilus provides a combination of DDS-1 (a high-quality acidophilus) with colustrum and fructooligosaccharides, which promote the growth of friendly bacteria in the body. This product also contains enzymes that break down proteins, fats and starches. The bacteria in Enzydophilus are freeze-dried to ensure they are alive when they reach the intestine and so every two capsules are guaranteed to contain 2.5 billion live bacteria.

Anti-Yeast Programme

Common factors associated with a yeast syndrome:
◆ Frequent or long-term use of antibiotics
◆ Use of birth-control pill
◆ Premenstrual syndrome
◆ Recurrent genital thrush in women and men
◆ Regular use of cortisone-based drugs
◆ Cravings for sweet foods, bread or alcohol
◆ Sensitivity to moulds and dampness
◆ Mental symptoms such as depression, mood swings or confusion
◆ Chronic fatigue, indigestion or food reactions
◆ Recurrent skin and/or nail fungus infections such as athlete's foot

Eight-week treatment plan

1. Do not feed the yeast on the foods upon which it thrives; follow the guidelines below for the next eight weeks.

Eat more of these foods		Avoid these foods	
Vegetables	Beans	All sugar	Baked foods
Meats	Nuts and seeds	Alcohol	Vinegar
Poultry	Butter	Fruit juice	Pickles
Eggs	Oils	Dried fruit	Cheese
Lemon	Refined flour	Mushrooms	Fish
Whole grains	Fresh fruit (two pieces per day only)	Breads	

2. Take the Candida Formula during the programme as follows:

Week 1	2 capsules between meals twice daily
Week 2	2 capsules between meals twice daily
Week 3	1 capsule between meals twice daily
Week 4	1 capsule between meals twice daily
Weeks 5–8	1 capsule between lunch and dinner only

3. Take a probiotic formula to re-establish the gut bacteria balance.

Suggested formula – Enzydophilus

Week 1	1 capsule taken three times daily with food
Week 2–8	1 capsule with a meal

❧ ROBERT'S COMPLEX ❧

The old naturopathic remedy Robert's Formula has a long history of use in inflammatory bowel disease, peptic ulcers and other causes of diarrhoea. Legend has it that a sailor named Robert had a severe peptic ulcer and every time he visited a new port he would add a new plant remedy to his self-made formula. Eventually, Robert healed his ulcer.

Enzymatic Therapy's version of this formula, Robert's Complex, contains niacinamide in a special blend of herbs and other natural factors. American cranesbill, cabbage, marshmallow, okra and slippery elm are rich in mucilage – a substance that forms a slippery mass when suspended in water. Robert's Complex also contains a duodenal substance to support the digestive system.

Mode of action
NIACINAMIDE: Necessary for carbohydrate, fat and protein

metabolism. Helps maintain health of skin, tongue and digestive system.

MARSHMALLOW EXTRACT: A demulcent (an oily or mucilaginous agent used to soothe or soften an irritated surface) with soothing properties on the mucous membranes.

ECHINACEA ROOT EXTRACT: An antibacterial that is also used to promote normalisation of the immune system.

AMERICAN CRANESBILL: A gastrointestinal haemostatic (a medicine or blood component that serves to stop bleeding).

GOLDENSEAL ROOT EXTRACT: Inhibits growth of many enteropathic (intestinal) bacteria.

SLIPPERY ELM: A demulcent (an oily or mucilaginous agent used to soothe or soften an irritated surface).

CABBAGE EXTRACT: Raw cabbage juice has been well documented as having remarkable success in treating peptic ulcers.

❦ DOCTOR'S CHOICE FOR DIABETICS ❦

Doctor's Choice for Diabetics is designed to provide an extra nutritional support for individuals with elevated blood sugar levels and should be used in conjunction with the Doctor's Choice gender-specific multiple and Doctor's Choice Flax Oil products.

Recommendations
Two tablets twice a day.

Ingredients

Amounts per 2 tablets		% Daily Value
Vitamin C (ascorbic acid)	300mg	500
Vitamin E (mixed tocopherols)	100iu	333
Vitamin B6 (pyridoxine HCI)	10mg	500
Folic acid	400mg	100
Vitamin B12 (cyanocobalamin)	400mg	6,667
Biotin	1,000mg	333
Magnesium (Krebs cycle chelate)	100mg	25
Zinc (picolinate)	7.5mg	50
Selenium (aspartate)	50 mg	71
Copper (picolinate)	0.5mg	25
Manganese (Krebs cycle chelate)	7.5mg	375
Chromium (picolinate)	200mg	167
Sodium	6mg	0.3

Gymnema sylvestre leaves extract (standardised to contain 24% gymnemic acid)	200mg	*
Bitter melon (*Momordica charantia*) (whole fruit extract)	200mg	*
Fenugreek (*Trigonella foenum-graecum*) (seed extract 4:1)	100mg	*
Bilberry (*Vaccinium myrtillus fructus*)	40mg	*
Mixed bioflavonoids (citrus)	25mg	*
Vanadyl sulfate	5mg	*

* Daily Value not established.

Other ingredients: calcium carbonate, cellulose, cellulose gum, silicon dioxide, dicalcium phosphate, magnesium stearate and calcium silicate.

Contains no sugar, salt, yeast, wheat, gluten, corn, dairy products, artificial colouring, artificial flavouring or preservatives.

❦ KREBS CYCLE CHELATES ❦

The complete multiple mineral dietary supplement.

Recommendations
Four tablets a day.

Warning
Accidental overdose of iron-containing products is a leading cause of fatal poisoning in children under six. Keep this product out of the reach of children. In case of accidental overdose, call your doctor or a poison control centre immediately.

Ingredients

Amount per 4 tablets	%	*Daily Value*
Calcium (ET-CFMSA)*	600mg	60
Iron (ET-CFMSA)*	5mg	28
Iodine (marine organic minerals)	100mg	67
Magnesium (ET-CFMSA)*	400mg	100
Zinc (ET-CFMSA)*	15mg	100
Selenium (ET-CFMSA)*	75mg	107
Copper (ET-CFMSA)*	1mg	50
Manganese (ET-CFMSA)*	2mg	100
Chromium (ET-CFMSA)*	100mg	83

Molybdenum (ET-CFMSA)*	25mg	33
Sodium	10mg	<1
Potassium (ET-CFMSA)*	99mg	3
Boron (ET-CFMSA)*	4mg	†
Vanadium (ET-CFMSA)*	50mg	†

* Enzymatic Therapy's bioactive minerals are chelated to the Krebs Cycle intermediates (citrate, fumarate, malate, succinate and alpha ketoglutarate). These organic acids are responsible for energy production within every cell of the body. Minerals chelated to the Krebs Cycle are better absorbed and utilised.

† Daily value not established.

Other ingredients: cellulose, cellulose gum, stearic acid, silicon dioxide, magnesium stearate and water-soluble film coating.

Contains no sugar, yeast, wheat, gluten, corn, soy, dairy products, artificial colouring, artificial flavouring or preservatives.

❧ PHYTO-BIOTIC ❧

Herbal dietary supplement with high concentrations of berberine.

Recommendations
Two capsules three times a day.

Ingredients
Amount per 2 capsules:

Barberry (*Berberis vulgaris*)	400mg*
(Bark of root extract 6:1)	
Oregon grape (*Berberis aquifolium*)	400mg*
(Root extract 6:1)	
Goldenseal (*Hydrastis canadensis*)	100mg*
(Root extract 4:1)	

Standardised to contain 5% total alkaloids including berberine, hydrastine and canadine.

* Daily Value not established.

Other ingredients: cellulose, magnesium stearate, silicon dioxide and gelatin capsule.

Contains no sugar, salt, yeast, wheat, gluten, corn, soy, dairy produces, artificial colouring, artificial flavouring or preservatives.

❧ SHIITAKE ❧

Common name: Hua gu. Wild shiitake mushrooms (*Lentinan edodes*) are native to Japan, China and other Asian countries and typically grow on fallen broadleaf trees. Shiitake is widely cultivated throughout the world, including the United States. The fruiting body is used medicinally.

Shiitake has been revered in Japan and China as both a food and medicinal herb for thousands of years. Wu Ri, a famous physician from the Chinese Ming dynasty (AD 1368–1644), wrote extensively about this mushroom, noting its ability to increase energy, cure colds and eliminate worms.

Supportive conditions
Chemotherapy support
Hepatitis support
HIV support

Active constituents
Shiitake contains proteins, fats, carbohydrates, soluble fibre, vitamins and minerals. In addition, shiitake's key ingredient – found in the fruiting body – is a polysaccharide called lentinan. Commercial preparations employ the powdered mycelium of the mushroom before the cap and stem grow; this is called LEM (lentinan edodes mycelium extract). LEM is also rich in polysaccharides and lignans.

Research indicates that LEM helps decrease chronic hepatitis B infectivity, as measured by specific liver and blood markers. A highly purified intravenous form of lentinan has been employed in Japan for the treatment of recurrent stomach cancer; it increases survival with this cancer (particularly when used in combination with chemotherapy). These effects may be due to shiitake's ability to stimulate specific types of white blood cells called T-lymphocytes. Case reports from Japan are also highly suggestive that lentinan is helpful in treating individuals with HIV infection. However, large-scale clinical trials have not yet been performed confirming this action.

Dosage information

The traditional intake of the whole, dried shiitake mushroom, in soups or as a decoction, is 6–16g a day. For LEM, the intake is 1–3g two or three times a day until the condition being treated improves. As LEM is the more concentrated and hence more potent extract, it is preferred over the crude mushroom. Tincture, in the amount of 2–4ml a day, can also be used.

Adverse reactions

Shiitake has an excellent record of safety but has been known to induce temporary diarrhoea and abdominal bloating when used in high dosages. Its safety during pregnancy has not yet been established.

❧ SLIPPERY ELM ❧

The slippery elm tree (*Ulmus rubra*) is native to North America, where it still primarily grows. The inner bark of the tree provides the greatest therapeutic benefit.

Native Americans found innumerable medicinal and other uses for this tree. Canoes, baskets and other household goods were made from the tree and its bark. Slippery elm was also used internally for everything from sore throats to diarrhoea. As a poultice it was considered a remedy for almost any skin condition.

Supportive conditions

Common cold/sore throat
Cough
Crohn's disease
Gastritis

LAMBERTS

Lamberts Healthcare is one of the finest companies in the market, providing top-quality products. Although they supply mainly vitamins, minerals and trace elements, they have a few herbal products which I am very happy to recommend, as some people prefer tablets to drops. (I still, however, feel that fresh herbal extracts are the best.) Most Lamberts products are formulated to meet European pharmaceutical standards (15 minutes' disintegration time for uncoated tablets, 30 minutes for coated tablets) or will disintegrate in less than one hour. The exception is time-release tablets, which are formulated to release their contents gradually over a period of six to eight hours, thus maximising tissue saturation.

Disintegrants are substances that produce a 'matrix' throughout the tablet that can be acted upon by the fluids in the digestive system. The disintegrants do not require acid conditions to work and all-out disintegration tests are carried out in pure water.

NELSONS

Nelsons has had a terrific impact not only on the British market but all over the world. Its products are trusted and I have not only prescribed them but also promoted them for many years. The pharmacy in Duke Street, London, is well worth a visit.

Nelsons is one of the oldest homoeopathic companies in Britain. It was in 1860 that a young pharmacist, Ernst Louis Ambrecht, came to London and opened a homoeopathic pharmacy in Ryder Street, where he could put into practice the principles he had learned from his teacher, Samuel Hahnemann, the father of homoeopathy. The business soon outgrew its premises and in 1890 it was moved to Duke Street, where it remains today. Ernst was succeeded by his son Nelson, who changed the name of the company to A. Nelson & Co.

Nelsons Formulated Range

Nelsons Formulated Range combines a number of remedies to create a range of products that offer easy-to-take relief for everyday illnesses. It has been designed with the first-time user in mind and offers an effective and non-drowsy alternative to conventional drug-based medication.

NOCTURA: Nelsons Noctura contains a unique selection of homoeopathic remedies, specifically combined to bring soothing relief from insomnia. A bad night's sleep is often the result of stress; a refreshing, natural night's sleep will help reduce that stress.

POLLENNA: Nelsons Pollenna contains a selection of homoeopathic remedies, specifically combined to protect from the distressing symptoms of hay fever and bring fast, effective relief. Pollenna does not cause drowsiness and can be taken with other medications.

TRAVELLA: Nelsons Travella contains a selection of homoeopathic remedies specifically combined to bring soothing relief from the unpleasant symptoms associated with travel sickness.

COLDENZA: Nelsons Coldenza is a homoeopathic remedy specifically designed to protect from the symptoms of cold and flu and bring fast, effective relief. For best results take immediately at the onset of flu or the early stages of a cold; keep warm and drink plenty of fluids. Coldenza does not cause drowsiness and can be taken with other medicines.

RHEUMATICA: Nelsons Rheumatica is a homoeopathic remedy specifically designed to bring effective relief from the symptomatic aches and pains associated with rheumatism, lumbago and sciatica.

CANDIDA: Nelsons Candida contains a specific homoeopathic remedy which stimulates natural resistance to the challenges of flora imbalances in the body. Candida is most effective when used in association with a diet management programme. Candida can be safely used in association with topical solutions to relieve immediate discomfort.

TEETHA: Nelsons Teetha is a homoeopathic remedy specifically designed to bring gentle, soothing relief to the painful symptoms of teething, thus calming both mother and baby. Teetha comes in an easy-to-administer granule form.

SOOTHA: Sootha cough syrup is a pleasant-tasting, soothing homoeopathic remedy. It contains Bryonia 6c, honey and lemon juice – natural ingredients that help to bring gentle relief to coughs in both adults and children of all ages.

TOOTHPASTE: Nelsons have developed a toothpaste specifically for users of homoeopathic medicine, the use of which will not interfere with delicate remedies.

POTTER'S

Potter's is another company with which I have worked for many years. It is the oldest herbal business in Britain, having been opened by Henry Potter in London in 1812. Since then, the name Potter's has been synonymous with all that is best in herbal medicine.

With the development of chemical drugs over the last century, there was a tendency for herbal medicine to be regarded as outdated and ineffective, and it is only in the last ten years or so that it has enjoyed a major revival and is now widely regarded as an important weapon in the armoury of health care. Of course, many chemical medicines are now based on ingredients synthesised from plants, but in herbal medicines the whole herb is used. This is because herbal experts believe that many components of the plant are synergistic and so using the whole herb enhances its healing properties. Another important distinction between chemical drugs and herbal medicines is that the latter are designed to work by treating the underlying causes of a problem rather than just alleviating the symptoms.

Today all medicines, including herbals, must be licensed by the Medicines Control Agency. The law is continually being tightened to root out products which claim or imply medicinal benefits while avoiding the licensing process and it is likely that these will need to conform or they will disappear from the shelves. From the retailer's point of view, then, it is vital to concentrate only on genuine medicines which can be stocked and recommended with confidence. Herbal medicines can be prescribed and reimbursed on the same terms as other medicines and more and more GPs are now doing just that, finding them particularly useful for long-standing or recurring conditions where possible dependency or side effects may have to be considered.

In most of Europe, herbal medicines have been regarded for many years as mainstream medicines and are sold alongside drugs in pharmacies everywhere. The market for herbals is vast as they are universally recognised as having a useful and important place in medical treatment. As the UK herbal medicine market continues to expand, retailers owe it to their customers to be well stocked with, and well informed about, these gentle alternatives to chemical drugs.

As with any medicine, care should be taken to read the label, particularly regarding dosage instructions and cautions. Some herbal remedies – like any medicinal products – are not suitable for pregnant women or young children. Where a patient is already taking prescribed medicine, a doctor should be consulted before stopping that treatment, and should also be advised when additional over-the-counter remedies – herbal or chemical – are taken.

Over-the-counter herbal medicines are generally known for being free from unwelcome side effects but, again, if a patient notices any problems, the advice is to stop taking the product and consult a health professional.

Customers new to herbal preparations may be concerned about whether a product is 'proper medicine'. They will be reassured to learn that herbal medicines are licensed by the Medicines Control Agency – which also licenses chemical drugs – and that they must meet strict standards of efficacy, quality and safety. A herbal medicine – distinct from any other herbal product – carries a PL number on the pack. And, of course, herbal remedies made by Potter's have the additional safeguard that they have been tried and tested over several generations of satisfied customers.

Potter's Licensed Medicines are:
◆ ACIDOSIS (tablets and oral liquid) Indigestion
◆ ADIANTINE (external liquid) Poor hair conditions, dandruff
◆ ANASED (tablets) Headaches and other pain
◆ ANTIBRON (tablets) Coughs
◆ ANTIFECT (tablets) Hay fever, blocked sinuses, catarrh
◆ ANTIGLAN (tablets) Male urinary problems
◆ ANTITIS (tablets) Female urinary problems
◆ APPETISER (oral liquid) Loss of appetite
◆ BACKACHE (tablets and oral liquid) Backache caused by over-exertion
◆ BALM OF GILEAD (oral liquid) Coughs (especially in children)
◆ BOLDEX (tablets) Slimming
◆ CATARRH MIXTURE (oral liquid) Catarrh in the nose and throat
◆ CHEST MIXTURE (oral liquid) Coughs and catarrh
◆ CHLOROPHYLL (tablets) Temporary tiredness
◆ COMFREY OINTMENT Bruises and strains
◆ DERMACREME (ointment) Minor cuts, grazes and burns
◆ DIURETABS (tablets) Periodic fluid retention
◆ ECHINACEA (tablets and oral liquid) Susceptibility to infection

- ECZEMA OINTMENT Irritation and itching from eczema
- ELDERFLOWER, PEPPERMINT WITH COMPOSITION ESSENCE (oral liquid) Colds, chills
- ELIXIR OF BLACK HAW AND GOLDENSEAL (oral liquid) Menopausal flooding
- ELIXIR OF DAMIANA AND SAW PALMETTO (oral liquid) Loss of energy in older males
- GARLIC (tablets) Colds and catarrh
- G.B. (tablets) Temporary discomfort after eating
- HERBHEAL (ointment) Skin irritation
- HOREHOUND AND ANISEED COUGH MIXTURE (oral liquid) Coughs
- INDIAN BRANDEE (oral liquid) Digestive discomfort
- INDIGESTION MIXTURE (oral liquid) Heartburn, flatulence and indigestion
- JAMAICAN SARSAPARILLA (oral liquid) Minor skin problems
- KAS-BAH HERB (infusion) Temporary urinary and bladder discomfort
- LIFE DROPS (oral liquid) Flu, colds and chills
- LIGHTNING COUGH REMEDY (oral liquid) Coughs
- LION CLEANSING HERB (tablets and infusion) Occasional constipation
- MALTED KELP (tablets) Convalescence, also rheumatic pain
- NEWRELAX (tablets) Tenseness and irritability
- NINE RUBBING OILS (external liquid) Muscular pain and stiffness
- NODOFF (tablets and oral liquid) Sleeping problems
- OUT OF SORTS (tablets) Occasional constipation
- PEERLESS COMPOSITION ESSENCE (oral liquid) Colds and chills
- PEGINA (oral liquid) Colds and chills
- PILETABS (tablets) Haemorrhoid discomfort
- PREMENTAID (tablets) Periodic bloating feeling
- PROTAT (oral liquid) Bladder discomfort in males
- PSORASOLV (ointment) Mild psoriasis
- RASPBERRY LEAF (tablets) Menstrual cramps
- RHEUMATIC PAIN (tablets) Aches and pains of rheumatism
- ROSEMARY, MEDICATED EXTRACT OF (external liquid) Poor hair condition
- ST JOHN'S WORT COMPOUND (oral liquid) A pharmacy-only product
- SCIARGO (tablets) Sciatica and lumbago
- SENNA (tablets) Occasional constipation

- ◆ SKIN CLEAR (tablets) Minor skin conditions and blemishes
- ◆ SKIN CLEAR (ointment) Mild acne and dry eczema
- ◆ SKIN ERUPTIONS MIXTURE (oral liquid) Mild eczema, psoriasis
- ◆ SLIPPER ELM (tablets) Convalescence
- ◆ SPANISH TUMMY MIXTURE (oral liquid) Non-persistent diarrhoea
- ◆ STOMACH MIXTURE (oral liquid) Stomach ache and upsets
- ◆ STRENGTH (tablets) Convalescence
- ◆ TABRITIS (tablets) Rheumatic pain and stiffness
- ◆ VALERIAN FORMULA (tablets) Stresses and strains of modern life
- ◆ VARICOSE OINTMENT Irritation from varicosity
- ◆ VEGETABLE COUGH REMOVER (oral liquid) Coughs
- ◆ WATERSHED (tablets and oral liquid) Fluid retention
- ◆ WELLWOMAN (tablets) Problems in female middle age

Some of my favourite Potter's remedies are:

🦋 ACIDOSIS 🦋

Active ingredients
EACH TABLET CONTAINS: Meadowsweet 160mg; charcoal medicinal vegetable BPC 1934 40mg; rhubarb BP 5 mg. Also contains: sucrose, dextrose monochydrate, Providone 30, cinnamon, cardamon seed, talc, starch, aniseed oil, caraway oil and magnesium stearate.

Meadowsweet is an astringent, antacid and stomachic. Charcoal absorbs toxic matter. Rhubarb is an astringent stomachic.

Dosage information
ADULTS: Two tablets three times a day after meals. For best results take regularly for several weeks.
CHILDREN: Not applicable.

🦋 ANASED 🦋

Active ingredients
EACH TABLET CONTAINS: Hops 30mg; Jamaica dogwood 90mg; dry extract wild lettuce 5:1 54mg; dry extract passiflora 5:1

36mg; dry extract pulsatilla 3:1 15mg. Also contains: sucrose, lactose, sodium starch glycollate, talc, magnesium stearate, shellac, kaolin light, titanium dioxide, black and yellow iron oxides.

Hops is sedative, relaxant and a diuretic and induces sleep in higher dosage. Dogwood Jamaica is sedative and painkilling. Wild lettuce is a mild sedative.

Dosage information
ADULTS: One or two tablets three times a day and two at bedtime. Not for children.

❦ ANTIFECT ❦

Active ingredients
EACH TABLET CONTAINS: Garlic 30mg; garlic oil 1mg; dry extract Echinacea 10:22 13.2mg. Also contains: charcoal medicinal vegetable, sucrose, acacia, stearic acid, talc, magnesium stearate, croscarmellose, silica, gelatin, calcium carbonate light, titanium dioxide, black and yellow iron oxides.

Garlic and its oil are antimicrobial, anticatarrhal and expectorant. Echinacea acts against infections, is anti-inflammatory and stimulates the immune system.

Dosage information
ADULTS: Two tablets three times a day.
CHILDREN: Over eight, half the adult dose. Not for children under eight.

❦ CLEANING HERB TABLETS ❦

Active ingredients
EACH TABLET CONTAINS: Senna leaves tinnevelly BP 100mg; aloes (Cape) BP 45mg; cascara bark BP 30mg; dandelion root 30mg; fennel seed 15mg. Also contains: dicalcium phosphate, sucrose, talc, magnesium stearate and sodium starch glycollate.

Senna leaves, aloes and cascara bark are purgative. Dandelion root stimulates the liver and increases bile production. Fennel seed is carminative and reduces griping pains due to purgatives.

Dosage information
ADULTS: One or two tablets at bedtime when necessary. Not for children.

❧ RASPBERRY LEAF ❧

Active ingredients
EACH TABLET CONTAINS: Dried aqueous extractive (4:1) from raspberry leaf 113mg. Also contains: sucrose, lactose, starch, cocoa, acacia, talc and magnesium stearate.

Raspberry leaves are astringent with a specific action on muscles of the uterus.

Dosage information
ADULTS ONLY: Two tablets after each meal.

❧ SLIPPERY ELM ❧

Active ingredients
EACH TABLET CONTAINS: Slippery elm bark 400mg; cinnamon, clove and peppermint oils 0.001ml each. Also contains: sucrose, acacia, silica, magnesium stearate and stearic acid.

Slippery elm is soothing and protective to the lining of the stomach and intestines. Cinnamon, clove and peppermint oils relieve stomach gas.

Dosage information
ADULTS ONLY: One or two tablets up to five times a day to be chewed after each meal.

❧ CLEANSING HERB ❧

Active ingredients
Blended herb containing Buckthorn bark (frangula) 8 per cent; Psyllium seeds light 12 per cent w/w; senna leaves tinnevelly BP 50 per cent w/w. Also contains: elderflowers, fennel seed and mate.

Senna leaf and Buckthorn bark are purgative. Psyllium seeds are a bulk laxative. Fennel seeds are carminative.

Dosage information
ADULTS: Half a level teaspoonful night or morning when required. Vary the dose as required. Place the herb in a mug; add boiling water. Allow to stand for 15 minutes; then drink the lot.

❦ TABRITIS ❦

Active ingredients
EACH TABLET CONTAINS: Elderflowers 60mg; prickly ash bark 60mg; yarrow 75mg; dry extract burdock root 100:37 22mg; dry extract clivers 100:28 17mg; dry extract poplar bark 10:16 16mg; dry extract uva-ursi 5:2 24mg. Also contains: dry extract senna leaf, sucrose, acacia, dextrose monohydrate, talc, maize starch, alginic acid, magnesium stearate and ethyl cellulose.

Elderflowers induce perspiration. Prickly ash bark stimulates the circulation. Yarrow is anti-inflammatory. Dry extract burdock root and dry extract clivers are eliminatory. Dry extract poplar bark is antirheumatic and a weak painkiller. Dry extract uva-ursi is diuretic.

Dosage information
ADULTS: Two tablets three times a day. Not recommended for children.

❦ VARICOSE OINTMENT ❦

Active ingredients
Cade oil BPC 2.3 per cent w/w; Hamamelis water BPC 7.4 per cent w/w; zinc oxide BP 3.57 per cent w/w. Also contains: emulsifying wax, wood alcohols, hard paraffin, butylated hydroxyanisole, iron oxide colourants and yellow soft paraffin.

Cade oil breaks keratin in skin cells and reduces the itch. Witch hazel is astringent. Zinc oxide is astringent and gives soothing protection.

Dosage information
ADULTS: Apply to affected parts morning and evening. Not for children.

❧ GINKGO BILOBA 2000 ❧

Presentation
A brown speckled coated tablet. Each tablet delivers:
◆ Standardised extract (50:1) of *Ginkgo biloba* leaves 40mg providing flavonglycosides 9.6mg and ginkgolides A, B, C and bilobalide 2.4mg.
◆ Tableted with: microcrystalline cellulose, dicalcium phosphate, crosslinked sodium carboxymethylcellulose, stearic acid, magnesium stearate, silicon dioxide, hydroxypropylmethyl cellulose, magnesium silicate and carnauba wax.
◆ Disintegration time: less than one hour.

Uses
Originating in China, *Ginkgo biloba*, also known as the ginkgo tree, is the world's oldest living tree species. Its longevity is attributed to its ability to withstand insects, disease and pollution due to the pharmaceutically active compounds in its leaves. The Chinese have long taken *Ginkgo biloba*, particularly the elderly.

Ginkgo extract is obtained solely from the leaves, which contain flavonols glycosides, flavonoids, diterpenes, plant sterols and organic acids. Extensive studies have been conducted using a standardised extract called Ginkgo Biloba Extract (GBE), with a content of 24 per cent glycosides. This compound, sourced in Japan, is rich in bioflavonoids, which are thought to help maintain the integrity of capillary walls.

Ginkgo helps to maintain the circulation of the blood which:
◆ helps keep hands and feet warm
◆ helps maintain the brain's oxygen supply, and thus
◆ helps maintain brain function.

Ginkgo Biloba Extract is also available as a one-a-day, high-potency time release product (see below).

Usage and administration
One to three tablets a day after a meal, or as directed by practitioner.

Contra-indications/warnings
This supplement should not be taken by pregnant or breastfeeding women.

Adverse reactions
None known at the recommended usage.

Pharmaceutical precautions
To be stored in a cool, dry place and protected from light.

Legal category
Food supplement.

🦋 SILICA 🦋

Presentation
A hard gelatin capsule. Each capsule delivers:
Powdered bamboo gum (*Bambousa arundinacea*) 320mg
   providing silica 200mg.
Encapsulated with: gelatin and magnesium stearate.

Uses
This product has been sourced from Europe's leading herbal company based in France and provides bamboo gum. Bamboo gum is rich in compounds called glycosaminoglycans, containing a constituent of structurally strong tissues such as arteries, tendons, skin, connective tissue and the cornea of the eye. Human glycosaminoglycans are involved with maintaining normal regulation of cholesterol levels and with the normal heart, brain and peripheral circulation, as well as being components of bone, cartilage and aortic tissue.

Usage and administration
One capsule three times a day with a meal, or as directed by practitioner.

Contra-indications/warnings
None known at the recommended usage.

Adverse reactions
None known at the recommended usage.

Pharmaceutical precautions
To be stored in a cool, dry place and protected from light.

Legal category
Food supplement.

❦ COLLADEEN (Anthocyanidin Complex) ❦

Presentation
A hard gelatin capsule. Each capsule delivers:

Anthocyanidin (from extracts of bilberry, cranberry and grape seed) 80mg.

Encapsulated with: microcrystalline cellulose, dicalcium phosphate, gelatin, magnesium stearate and silicon dioxide.

Uses
Anthocyanidins (also known as OPCs and pycnogenols or leucocyanidins) are similar in structure to bioflavonoids but are believed by many researchers to be much more bioactive. This is likely to be due to their high solubility, which enables them to be well absorbed and dispersed throughout the body with ease. As antioxidants, they are active in lipid as well as water environments, a unique nature of these plant pigments. They are up to 15 times more powerful than vitamin E. They are also known to support the many areas of the body containing collagen and to help with anti-inflammatory processes.

Anthocyanidins have been the subject of a great deal of scientific work, much of it concerned with their role with collagen, which is the elastic-like material found in certain tissues. In particular, collagen is found in high concentrations in capillary walls and in Europe people often choose to take anthocyanidins on a regular basis to help maintain the health of their peripheral circulation. Collagen is also responsible for the suppleness and firmness of the skin and it has long been recognised that skin health and complexion is influenced to a great degree by dietary factors.

Lamberts Colladeen uses three rich sources of anthocyanidins. The anthocyanidins are obtained from the plant material in an extraction process that greatly concentrates these active components, in some cases by up to 500 times their level in the original plant material.

Usage and administration
One or two capsules daily with a meal, or as directed by

practitioner. It should be noted that Colladeen will be reformulated as tablets during the year 2000.

Contra-indications/warnings

This supplement should not be taken by pregnant or breastfeeding women.

Adverse reactions

None known at the recommended usage.

Pharmaceutical precautions

To be stored in a cool, dry place and protected from light.

Legal category

Food supplement.

❧ PYCNOGENOL (Pine Bark Extract) ❧

Presentation

A hard gelatin capsule. Each capsule delivers:
Pine bark extract (Pycnogenol) 20mg
Encapsulated with: microcrystalline cellulose, gelatin, magnesium stearate and silicon dioxide.

Uses

Pycnogenol is a remarkable herbal extract with the unique primary ingredient known as proanthocyanidin, which in molecular structure is similar to flavonoids. Its unique action, however, is due to its bioavailability and non-toxicity.

Pyconogenol first came to be researched by Dr Jack Masquelier of the University of Bordeaux, France, after he read of an unknown substance being used successfully by members of an expedition. His research concentrated on the naturally derived proanthocyanidins in Pycnogenol, which are found to have supreme effects as antioxidants. *In vitro* testing shows Pycnogenol has powerful antioxidant properties like those of vitamins C and E.

As a consequence of Dr Masquelier's findings, he developed the pine bark extraction process and was awarded a US patent for the use of Pycnogenol as a free radical scavenger. Studies have confirmed its antioxidant effects when two capsules a day are taken.

Usage and administration
One or two capsules daily with a meal, or as directed by practitioner.

Contra-indications/warnings
This supplement should not be taken by pregnant women.

Adverse reactions
None known at the recommended usage.

Pharmaceutical precautions
To be stored in a cool, dry place and protected from light.

Legal category
Food supplement.

🦋 COD LIVER OIL 🦋

Presentation
A soft gelatin capsule. Each capsule delivers:

Cod liver oil	1,000mg	
providing omega-3	258mg	
of which EPA and DHA	207mg	
Vitamin A	800ug	(2,664iu)
Vitamin D	5ug	(200iu)
Vitamin E	10ug	(15iu)

Encapsulated with: gelatin and glycerin.

Uses
The parent acid in the omega-3 family of polyunsaturates is alpha-linolenic acid, which can be converted in the body to longer chain members such as eicosapentaenoic acid (EPA) and docosahexaenoic acid (DHA). EPA may help keep the heart healthy by maintaining normal blood lipid levels, normal platelet function and via the production of eicosanoids (prostaglandins and leukotrienes) maintain optimum joint health, whilst DHA is believed to play an important role in the transmission of electrical impulses across synapses in the brain. The main dietary sources of omega-3 fatty acids are fatty fish, which are little consumed by Western populations.

The Inuit were found to have lower levels of low-density lipoproteins (LDL) and higher levels of high-density lipoproteins (HDL). Fatty acids in fish oils consumed by the Inuit are thought to be the reason why they can eat such a high-fat diet and yet maintain a healthy heart.

Cod liver oil provides omega-3 fatty acids as well as vitamins which maintain normal growth and healthy hair, skin and nails. Individuals including teenagers who rely on fast snack foods or those who are housebound and get little sunlight, and growing children, are amongst those who may choose this supplement.

Usage and administration
One capsule daily with a meal, or as directed by practitioner.

Contra-indications/warnings
USE IN PREGNANCY: Vitamin A supplements should not exceed 2,664iu (800ug) daily, except on the advice of a doctor or ante-natal clinic.

Adverse reactions
Over-usage: Prolonged ingestion of massive amounts of vitamins A and D can lead to hypervitaminosis states. Symptoms include a dry mouth, rough skin, painful joint swellings, anorexia and vomiting. These disappear when supplementation is discontinued.

Pharmaceutical precautions
To be stored in a cool, dry place and protected from light.

Legal category
Food supplement.

❦ CRANBERRY COMPLEX POWDER ❦

Presentation
A pink soluble powder. Each 5g delivers:
Vitamin C   60mg
Cranberry powder   2,470mg
Fructo-oligosaccharides   2,470mg
Other ingredients: magnesium hydroxide and tricalcium phosphate.

Uses
Cranberry juice has long been known to women for its ability

to help maintain the health of the urinary system. However, cranberry juice is very sharp to the taste and consequently commercial cranberry drinks are laden with sugar and high in calories.

Lamberts Cranberry Complex is produced from fresh mature cranberries, which are first washed and depectinised to remove unwanted substances. The juice is then dehydrated at low temperature and low pressure and spray-dried to produce a sugar-free concentrate. This ensures that the unique properties of cranberries may be enjoyed by those following sugar-restricted diets. Approximately 25 grams of fresh cranberries are used to produce just one gram of concentrate.

Cranberry Complex is mixed with a complex carbohydrate called fructo-oligosaccharide (FOS), a sweet, easily dissolved substance extracted from chicory root. FOS acts as a probiotic, which means it encourages the growth of friendly bacteria, which help to suppress pathogenic, troublesome bacteria.

Usage and administration
Five to ten grams daily, or as directed by practitioner.

Contra-indications/warnings
None known at the recommended usage.

Adverse reactions
None known at the recommended usage.

Pharmaceutical precautions
To be stored in a cool, dry place and protected from light.

Legal category
Food supplement.

ECHINACEA

Presentation
A hard gelatin capsule. Each capsule delivers:
Echinacea purpurea equivalent to 1,000mg (as 200mg of a 5:1 extract) providing 4 per cent phenolic compounds.
Encapsulated with: gelatin, microcrystalline cellulose, magnesium stearate and silicon dioxide.

Uses

Echinacea purpurea, also known as purple coneflower, is widely used on the continent. It is one of the most well-researched herbs available, with many published reports demonstrating its active properties.

Echinacea is rich in numerous important constituents. Organic phenolic compounds present include echinacoside (a caffeic acid derivative), cichoric acid (particularly high in *Echinacea purpurea* compared to other species), chlorogenic acid and cynarin.

Although analysis of *Echinacea purpurea* has yielded an array of chemical constituents with some pharmacological activity, it is the organic phenolic compounds that are used for standardisation procedures.

Standardised extracts are favoured by Lamberts since the extraction and concentration procedures ensure that the herbal product is far more potent than those products based on a powdered whole herb, where no attempt is made to concentrate the active ingredients. The 200mg extract is made from over 1,000mg of dried powder and is therefore likely to be five times stronger than a product containing simply 200mg of powdered plant material.

Usage and administration

One or two capsules daily with a meal, or as directed by practitioner. Echinacea is best taken for two- to three-week periods.

Contra-indications/warnings

This supplement should not be taken by pregnant or breastfeeding women.

Adverse reactions

None known at the recommended usage.

Pharmaceutical precautions

To be stored in a cool, dry place and protected from light.

Legal category

Food supplement.

❦ MILK THISTLE ❦

Presentation
A hard gelatin capsule. Each capsule delivers:
Milk thistle equivalent to 3,000mg (as 100mg of a 30:1 extract)
  providing Silymarin 70mg.
Encapsulated with: microcrystalline cellulose, gelatin,
magnesium stearate and silicon dioxide.

Uses
Silymarin is the active principal from the fruit of *Silybum
marianum*, better known as the milk thistle. It consists of three
isomers called silybin, silidanin and silicristin, which are all
classed as flavonolignans, silybin being the most important
constituent.

For centuries it has been thought that the herb could have
beneficial effects on maintaining the health of the liver, and
studies over the past 20 years have indicated that when
silymarin is taken orally, the active ingredients remain in the
liver. The daily job of the liver is to detoxify the blood of
harmful toxins taken in with foods, such as alcohol, pollutants
and bacteria. Silymarin has also been shown to have antioxidant
properties. Antioxidants help protect the tissues against the
damaging effects of excess free radicals.

This high-potency product is a standardised extract prepared
from the mature seeds from milk thistle flowerheads and has a
guaranteed level of 70mg silymarin.

Usage and administration
One capsule daily with a meal, or as directed by practitioner.

Contra-indications/warnings
This supplement should not be taken by pregnant or
breastfeeding women.

Adverse reactions
None known at the recommended usage.

Pharmaceutical precautions
To be stored in a cool, dry place and protected from light.

Legal category
Food supplement.

❧ SIBERIAN GINSENG ❧

Presentation
A hard gelatin capsule. Each capsule delivers:
Siberian ginseng equivalent to 1,500mg (as 100mg of a 15:1
    extract) providing Eleutheroside E 75ug Eleutheroside B
    150ug.
Encapsulated with: microcrystalline cellulose, gelatin,
magnesium stearate and silicon dioxide.

Uses
The name 'ginseng' can be applied to several plant products, all
of which consist of the roots of members of the Araliaceae
family. The use of Siberian ginseng (*Eleutherococcus senticosus*)
was developed by Russians seeking an alternative to the
Korean/Chinese ginseng (*Panax ginseng*).

Siberian ginseng is the world's best-known and most highly
researched adaptogen, helping the body to adapt to demanding
situations. The key constituents believed to be primarily
responsible for the plant's adaptogenic activity are a large group of
compounds called eleutherosides. It is these substances that are
used as markers in preparing a standardised extract because,
unlike *Panax ginseng*, Siberian ginseng does not contain
ginsenosides. For this reason it is regarded as a more gentle
preparation and, indeed, is often referred to as the female ginseng
by herbalists who believe it may be more applicable to women.

Lamberts Siberian Ginseng is a high-potency product best
taken early in the day, as its effect on sleep may be similar to that
of caffeine. Human studies involving long-term administration
of ginseng have involved ginseng-free periods of two to three
weeks every one to two months.

Usage and administration
One capsule daily, or as directed by practitioner.

Contra-indications/warnings
Unsuitable during pregnancy.

Adverse reactions
None known at the recommended usage.

Pharmaceutical precautions
To be stored in a cool, dry place and protected from light.

Legal category
Food supplement.

❧ HYPERICUM 136MG ❧

Presentation
A yellow, coated tablet. Each tablet delivers:
Hypericum equivalent to 1,360mg (as 170mg of an 8:1 extract) providing Hypericin 500ug.
Tableted with: microcrystalline cellulose, crosslinked sodium carboxymethylcellulose, magnesium stearate, stearic acid, silicon dioxide, hydroxypropylmethyl cellulose, colours: titanium dioxide and iron oxide, glycerin, magnesium silicate and carnauba wax.
Disintegration time: less than one hour.

Uses
St John's wort (*Hypericum perforatum*) is a perennial plant native to many parts of the world, including European countries and the USA. It prefers sunny areas and has numerous bright yellow flowers.

There has been a great deal of research published on standardised extracts of Hypericum. It has been a popular herb on the continent for hundreds of years and, in Germany alone, millions of supplements are sold every year. The key constituent to have received most attention is hypericin, and it is therefore this substance that is used as the standardisation marker in Lamberts extract.

Usage and administration
Two tablets daily, or as directed by practitioner.

Contra-indications/warnings
This supplement is not recommended for pregnant or breastfeeding women.

Adverse reactions
None known at the recommended usage.

Pharmaceutical precautions
To be stored in a cool, dry place and protected from light.

❦ VITEX AGNUS-CASTUS ❦

Presentation
A hard gelatin capsule. Each capsule delivers:
Vitex agnus-castus (as 100mg of a 10:1 extract) 1,000mg.
Encapsulated with: microcrystalline cellulose, dicalcium phosphate, magnesium stearate and silicon dioxide.

Uses
Vitex agnus-castus (often referred to as Vitex) is a shrub that originates from the Mediterranean. Some of the earliest scientific studies on Vitex for women's problems date back to 1954 in Germany. A recent survey among medical herbalists revealed strong support for the use of Vitex in the treatment of hormone imbalance syndromes among young and menopausal women.

Vitex berries are used in the manufacture of the herbal extract and contain a wide range of active compounds, including flavonoids and a group of compounds referred to as iridoids, which include aucubin and agnuside. Modern research has shown that the action of Vitex is at the highest level of hormonal control: the pituitary gland in the brain. Here, it is thought that Vitex mimics an important neurotransmitter referred to as dopamine, which helps to normalise the output of gonadotrophins that control sex hormones.

Vitex has been shown to help alleviate premenstrual symptoms, cycle irregularities and adverse menopausal symptoms.

Usage and administration
One capsule daily on rising, or as directed by practitioner.

Contra-indications/warnings
This supplement is not recommended for pregnant or breastfeeding women or for children.

Adverse reactions
None known at the recommended usage.

Pharmaceutical precautions
To be stored in a cool, dry place and protected from light.

Legal category
Food supplement.

❦ KAVA-KAVA ❦

Presentation
A film-coated tablet. Each tablet delivers:
Kava-kava (as 400mg extract) 2,000mg providing 30 per cent
  kavalactones 120mg.
Tableted with: dicalcium phosphate, microcrystalline cellulose,
crosslinked sodium carboxymethylcellulose, stearic acid, magnesium stearate, silicon dioxide, hydroxypropylmethyl cellulose,
colours: titanium dioxide and iron oxide and magnesium silicate.

Uses
Historically used for inducing a relaxing and calming effect,
kava-kava (*Piper methysticum*) extracts are still a popular choice
among practitioners today for those needing an anti-anxiety
preparation.

It is the large, branched rhizomes of the plant that the herbal
extracts are derived from. In fact, the kava rhizome is among the
few plant materials whose key active constituents are known
and well described. These are the kavalactones. Frequently
referred to as a 'nervine' tonic, kava-kava extracts are often used
for relatively short periods of time.

Usage and administration
One capsule daily, or as directed by practitioner.

Contra-indications/warnings
This supplement is not recommended for pregnant or
breastfeeding women or for children.

Adverse reactions
None known at the recommended usage.

Pharmaceutical precautions
To be stored in a cool, dry place and protected from light.

Legal category
Food supplement.

🦋 GINGER 🦋

Presentation
A soft gelatin capsule. Each capsule delivers:
Ginger root (as 120mg of a 100:1 extract) 12,000mg.
Encapsulated with: beeswax, sorbitan monolaurate, sunflower seed oil, gelatin, glycerin and colours: iron oxides.

Uses
Ginger is one of 1,400 species belonging to the *Zingiberaceae* family (other members include turmeric and cardamon). Ginger is the most popular of the family. It is a rhizome, although it is popularly referred to as 'root ginger'. It probably originated in the tropics and South-east Asia, but today it is the world's most widely cultivated spice. However, ginger is more than just a tasty spice. It is also known for its warming properties and is widely used as a digestive aid.

Usage and administration
One capsule daily, or as directed by practitioner.

Contra-indications/warnings
This supplement is not recommended for pregnant or breastfeeding women.

Adverse reactions
None known at the recommended usage.

Pharmaceutical precautions
To be stored in a cool, dry place and protected from light.

Legal category
Food supplement.

🦋 HYPERICUM 272MG 🦋

Presentation
An oval, yellow coated tablet. Each tablet delivers:
Hypericum equivalent to 2,720mg (as 340mg of an 8:1 extract) providing Hypericin 1,000ug.
Tableted with: dicalcium phosphate, microcrystalline cellulose, hydroxypropylmethylcellulose, colours: iron oxides and

titanium dioxide, magnesium silicate, crosslinked sodium carboxymethyl cellulose, silicon dioxide, magnesium stearate and stearic acid.

Usage and administration
One tablet daily, or as directed by practitioner.

Contra-indications/warnings
This supplement is not recommended for pregnant or breastfeeding women.

Adverse reactions
None known at the recommended usage.

Pharmaceutical precautions
To be stored in a cool, dry place and protected from light.

❧ SAW PALMETTO COMPLEX ❧

Presentation
A hard gelatin capsule. Two capsules deliver:

Beta carotene	12mg	
Equivalent to vitamin A	2,000ug	(6,600iu)
Vitamin E	68mg	
Vitamin C	300mg	
Thiamin (vitamin B1)	10mg	
Riboflavin (vitamin B2)	10mg	
Magnesium	15mg	
Zinc (as amino acid chelate)	15mg	
Glycine	140mg	
L-Glutamic acid	140mg	
L-Alanine	140mg	
Saw palmetto extract	320mg	

Encapsulated with: gelatin, microcrystalline cellulose, silicon dioxide, soya bean oil and magnesium stearate.

Uses
Saw palmetto (*Serenoa repens*) is a North American palm. Lamberts Saw Palmetto Complex contains the concentrated extract of the palm berries together with zinc and the antioxidant nutrients vitamin C, vitamin E and beta carotene.

In virtually all the studies carried out on saw palmetto, it is a concentrated extract that has been used (at 160mg extract twice daily), which is why Lamberts use an extract rather than just powdered berries that consist largely of fibre and sugars. The 160mg extract in each Saw Palmetto Complex capsule is equal to 1,920mg of powdered berry, i.e. 12 times stronger than the material used by many other manufacturers.

In addition to Saw Palmetto Complex, 1,000mg of Evening Primrose Oil daily is recommended to enhance the range of nutrients being added to the diet.

Usage and administration
Two capsules daily, or as directed by practitioner.

Contra-indications/warnings
None known at the recommended usage.

Adverse reactions
None known at the recommended usage.

Pharmaceutical precautions
To be stored in a cool, dry place and protected from light.

Legal category
Food supplement.

🦋 ALOE VERA 🦋

Presentation
A soft gelatin capsule. Each capsule delivers: Aloe vera juice equivalent to 10,000mg (as 50mg of a 20:1 extract).
Encapsulated with: soya bean oil, colours: titanium dioxide and chlorophyll, hydrogenated vegetable oil, beeswax and lecithin.

Uses
Aloe vera is the most widely known and used of over 300 aloe species, most of which are native to South Africa but centuries ago became widely distributed via the major trade routes.

Today, aloe vera is a popular house plant and the plant may be used in its simplest form by applying the gel topically. The gel is obtained simply by breaking the thick triangular leaves near their base and squeezing the fresh gel directly onto dry skin, abrasions or burns. The gel spoils quickly but can be made into an ointment, which can then be kept for longer-term use.

The juice comes from specialised cells beneath the thick outer skin of the leaves and contains a proportion of gel. Of the many historical uses for drinking aloe vera juice, the herb is best known for its effect in helping to maintain a healthy digestive system. However, the juice has a bitter taste and therefore a more convenient way to take the herb is in the form of capsules. Lamberts Aloe Vera capsules contain 50mg of concentrate equivalent to 10,000mg of fresh aloe vera juice.

Usage and administration
One or two capsules daily, or as directed by practitioner.

Contra-indications/warnings
None known at recommended usage. Best avoided during pregnancy.

Adverse reactions
None known at the recommended usage.

Pharmaceutical precautions
To be stored in a cool, dry place and protected from light.

Legal category
Food supplement.

POWER HEALTH

Power Health have nearly 30 years' experience in the herbal vitamin supplement market and manufacture a wide range of tablets and capsules. Popular products can be divided into four groups.

Core products include:
Cod liver oil: provides important omega-3 nutrients EPA and
   DHA.
Garlic: helps to maintain a healthy heart.
Evening primrose oil: the oil in the seed is rich in essential fatty
   acids, particularly gamma linolenic acid (GLA).
Vitamin C: important antioxidant.
Vitamin E: potent antioxidant.
Multivitamin: potent supplement with the added convenience
   of a single dosage.

Herbal products include:
St John's wort: the sunshine herb.
Echinacea: stimulates the immune system.
Kava-kava: to relieve anxiety.
Aloe vera: soothing properties.
Cranberry: helps maintain the health of the bladder.

Slimming range include:
Grapefruit pectin fibre: helps lower blood cholesterol.
Superleo: helps burn calories.
Calcium pyruvate: increases the metabolism, accelerating the
   burning of sugar and starch.
Chitosan and calcium: absorbs fat before it can be digested and
   expels it from the body.
Botanical Formula for Slimmers.

More specialised lines include:
MSM: organic sulphur.
Ginseng: a rejuvenating tonic which helps maintain health and
   vigour.
Royal Gellee: an excellent tonic with a rich combination of
   vitamins, minerals, amino acids and trace elements.
Glucosamine: helps maintain healthy cartilage, ligaments and
   tendons.
Mexican wild yam: has very high concentration of a substance

called diosgenin which is a form of natural progesterone.
Soya isoflavones, kudzo root and red clover: the isoflavones in
   soy have been well researched by scientists for their
   antioxidant and phytoestrogenic properties.

These Power Health products are the ones that I work with
most and they have given a lot of help to a great number of
people.

VITABIOTICS

Vitabiotics is a company which has some wonderful products. In my next book I shall write about them in more detail, but I want to mention Cardioace here. Cardioace is a new advanced formula for heart health. It is the only supplement in the UK to combine the benefits of omega-3 fatty acids with garlic, antioxidants and important trace minerals. The formula provides the nutritional building blocks for key enzymes in heart health, and ingredients thought to help maintain healthy blood cholesterol levels. It also includes nutrients which research has shown may be lower in those concerned with heart health.

The Cardioace formulation includes omega-3 fish oil, a rich source of EPA and DHA, which may play an important role in regulating blood pressure, cholesterol and triglyceride levels. Garlic is also included to help balance 'good' (high density) and 'bad' (low density) lipoproteins through its role in helping to decrease cholesterol production by the liver. Garlic may also help to maintain normal blood pressure. Further good news in heart nutrition has focused on vitamins B6, B12 and folic acid, which may work in synergy to help maintain healthy lower levels of a blood amino acid called homocysteine. High levels of homocysteine may be an independent risk factor for arteriosclerosis.

Vitamin E is thought to be beneficial for heart health through its key role in protecting fatty acids from oxidation. Lipids, or fats, travel around the body bound to complex spherical particles called lipoproteins. Low density lipoprotein (LDL) is what is commonly thought of as 'bad cholesterol', the main supplier of cholesterol to tissues. When LDL becomes oxidised, it gives rise to foam cells, one of the constituents in plaque. In order to get cholesterol back to the liver, where it can be excreted, a carrier molecule, or 'taxi', is required. High density lipoprotein (HDL) scavenges for free cholesterol in the tissues and transports it back to the liver. Oxidation of HDL, thought of as 'good cholesterol', interferes with its role in cholesterol transport. Antioxidants like vitamin E, along with vitamin C and selenium, help to prevent the oxidation of LDL and HDL, and may therefore be beneficial for heart health.

The Cardioace formulation is based on the very latest international findings on the role of nutrients in heart health, as well as numerous studies in the past 20 years. Backed up by almost 200 key references, Cardioace was developed with the help of leading scientists and with the input of the University of Reading, Department of Nutritional Science.

WELEDA

The Weleda company was founded in 1923 to manufacture medicines for the system of anthroposophical medicine developed by Rudolf Steiner.

Dr Rudolf Steiner (1861–1925) founded a school of scientific study which endeavours to go beyond the materialistic approach to science by developing the innate spiritual faculties of man. Through meditation and concentration these faculties may then be used to study the spiritual aspects of man, and their connections with the physical man on the one hand and the cosmos on the other. Steiner called this science 'anthroposophy'. By developing his own spiritual faculties, he evolved a philosophical doctrine, which he expounded in numerous lectures and books.

A group of doctors asked Steiner to establish the basis of an anthroposophically orientated medicine, and this he did in lectures and tutorials. Inspired by these courses, the doctors established a clinic near the headquarters of the anthroposophical movement in Dornach, Switzerland, under the direction of Steiner's principal medical collaborator, Dr Ita Wegman. With Dr Wegman, Dr Steiner wrote a short book on medicine called *Fundamentals of Therapy*, in which he outlined this approach to medicine.

Following these developments, the Weleda company was founded to manufacture new medicines and to prepare existing medicines according to special techniques developed by Dr Steiner and the physicians working with him. Branches now exist all over the world.

Weleda potencies are prepared by a special rhythmic method, which gives the remedy a dynamic effect beyond the simple homoeopathic potentisation. In addition, both the picking and the preparation of the remedies are related to the planetary movements as discovered by Dr Steiner in his spiritual scientific research. Cultivated remedies are grown by the bio-dynamic (organic) method and no effort is spared to prepare medicine of the highest quality.

Anyone wishing to find out more about Weleda products or anthroposophical medicine in general should contact Weleda directly or the Anthroposophical Society of Great Britain, Rudolf Steiner House, 35 Park Road, London NW1 6XT.

HERBAL AND HOMEOPATHIC
REMEDIES

This section lists 200 medical conditions and the fresh herb extracts and homoeopathic medicines that can be used to aid the body in the healing process. (Details of the herbal formulae, or combinations, suggested in the following pages are given in subsequent sections.) Before using this information, you should read the important points listed below.

Meanings of terms used
The terms '(1) Primary' and '(2) Secondary' are used for both the herb and homoeopathic categories. '(1) Primary' indicates the product (either herb or homoeopathic) that should be considered first; '(2) Secondary' indicates a product that can be used with a primary product.

Choosing and using a product
When choosing a product, first consider a formula (either herbal or homoeopathic). A formula will generally work better than a single herb or single homoeopathic remedy. A primary product can be used in combination with a secondary product or two primary products can be used in combination.

If herbal and homoeopathic products are being used together, they should not be taken at the same time. The homoeopathic product should be taken on an empty stomach (to improve effectiveness) and the herbal product taken at least an hour afterwards (the order can be reversed). Remember homoeopathic medicines should be taken with a clean mouth and empty stomach. This enhances their effect.

It's best to work with one condition at a time. If there are conditions that may be related (i.e. blood pressure and heart), you can work with both. The body works best when you work with one or two conditions at one time.

Herbal dosage

The usual dosage for herbs is 10–20 drops (undiluted or in a littler water or juice) three or four times a day. For herbal tablets, the dosage is one to three tablets three or four times a day. The dosage will need to be tailored to requirements. A child's dosage (under 60 lb) should be half the adult amount.

Homoeopathic dosage

The usual dosage for homoeopathic medicine is 10–20 drops or two to four tablets (taken under the tongue and held there for a few minutes) three or four times a day. Tablets should be completely dissolved under the tongue. The medicine should be taken with a clean, rinsed mouth (not contaminated with food, tobacco, toothpaste, etc.) and empty stomach (15–30 minutes before eating or at least an hour after eating). Also camphor, caffeine and mint or products that contain these elements sould be avoided. This will help the medicine to be more effective. In acute cases, the homoeopathic medicine can be taken as often as every hour. Some people may be sensitive under the tongue when using an alcohol-based homoeopathic medicine. There is nothing wrong with the product. When taking the medicine they should just open the mouth and drop the drops on the tongue. Then let the medicine mix with the saliva and hold it under the tongue for a few minutes. The medicine may also be mixed in a tablespoon of water and put under the tongue. The homoeopathic medicine should be taken until a day or two after the symptoms subside. Some of the homoeopathic medicines are available in tablet form. A child's dosage (under 60 lb) should be half the adult amount.

Final note about homoeopathy

Some people may experience a slight worsening or aggravation of symptoms for a short time. In acute cases (illnesses of short duration with severe rapid onset of symptoms, e.g. colds, flu, etc.) these symptoms may last four to eight hours. In chronic conditions (illnesses of longer duration, e.g. arthritis, menopause) a slight worsening of symptoms may last one to two weeks after beginning the medication. They should not give up but keep taking the homoeopathic product. This is a positive sign that the medicine is working.

Use herbs or homoeopathy?

The question sometimes comes up: 'When should I use a herbal

product and when should I use a homoeopathic product?'
Frankly, it's entirely up to the individual and what his or her
preferences may be. Here are a few pointers. For homoeopathic
medicines, instructions must be followed carefully (as to how to
take them) to provide the best results, whereas herbs you can
generally be taken just before or after a meal; also, the mouth
doesn't need to be rinsed clean as it does with homoeopathic
medicines. Homoeopathic medicines sometimes work faster
than herbs, but herbs sometimes work for a wider range of
people. Again, it all comes down to personal preference.

CLEANSING AND DETOXIFICATION PROGRAMME

One of the best things that we can do for our bodies as a 'whole' is to cleanse and detoxify it internally. The body is a dynamic unit, all parts working together in internal harmony to keep us going day after day. When we begin to feel sluggish and not able to do things as well as we usually can, or when we don't feel as good as we did in the past, it may be time for cleaning up our body and getting it on the right track again. The following five herbal formulae provide a thorough cleansing, regulating and rejuvenating programme which has been called a Rasayana Kalpa or 'Life Extension Programme' by Hindu physicians. In this programme the glands of the body that produce external secretions are stimulated so strongly that during the first three days they may produce some loose bowel movements. The functioning of the liver, gallbladder and bile duct are strongly stimulated. The kidneys also receive a thorough cleansing and are stimulated and regulated. A strong emphasis on good nutrition will help ensure that digestion improves and that the interrelationship of liver, kidney, gallbladder, intestine and stomach is normalised.

❦ ALOE–MYRRH–COLA NUT COMBINATION ❦

CONDITIONS: Stimulates proper digestion of the food and tones the stomach and intestinal tract. Useful for motion sickness.

DOSE: 10–15 drops in a little water, apple juice or rose hip tea, morning and evening.

CONTENTS: Aloe, cola nut, Peruvian bark, bitter orange, sweet myrtle, yellow gentian, myrrh, frankincense.

COMMENTS: This herbal formula affects the stomach by regulating and calming the stomach nerves. This in turn creates the ideal conditions for proper digestion. Due to its effect on the stomach nerves it is also an excellent remedy for the prevention of nausea and motion sickness.

❦ SENNA–BUCKTHORN–ALOE COMBINATION ❦

CONDITIONS: Blood cleanser and purifier. Stimulates function of intestines. As a laxative it stimulates elimination without becoming habit-forming. This combination also acts as a mild diuretic.

DOSE: Two tablets twice daily (morning and evening) with the aloe–myrrh–cola nut combination.

CONTENTS: Senna leaves, buckthorn bark, aloe, uva-ursi, fennel, chicory, blessed thistle, fumitory, dwarf elder, rest harrow, wild ginger, elecampane.

COMMENTS: This formula affects the functioning of the glands in the intestines and can be used in place of harmful laxatives. Due to the stronger secretion of the glands, the functioning of the intestines is stimulated. Should stronger stimulation be indicated, take three to four tablets, which will be sufficient for most cases. For children it is generally enough to crush one tablet and give it to the child mixed into juice or cereal. The nice part about this formula is that it is not habit-forming, and after it has been taken for a period of time it brings lasting results as long as sensible nutritional habits are maintained.

❧ SAFFRON–ALOE–CENTAURY COMBINATION ❧

CONDITIONS: Stimulates liver and gallbladder. Increases secretion of bile in cases of liver dysfunction.

DOSE: Three to five tablets with a glass of water (after lunch).

CONTENTS: Saffron, aloe, centaury, dandelion root, quackgrass, sarsaparilla, barberry.

COMMENTS: This herbal formula has a soothing as well as a stimulating effect on the liver and gallbladder. Since the secretions of bile will increase, it is of utmost importance to first take care of the proper function of the intestines (using the senna–buckthorn–aloe combination). In cases of chronic or stubborn constipation, it is recommended that you do not begin taking the saffron–aloe–centaury combination until proper bowel function is achieved.

❧ GOLDEN ROD–SILVERWEED–BIRCH COMBINATION ❧

CONDITIONS: Stimulates kidney and bladder function. Useful for kidney and bladder problems and increases urinary discharge.

DOSE: Along with the golden rod–birch–knotgrass combination tea, take five to ten drops of this formula in a little water three times a day.

CONTENTS: Golden rod (European), silverweed, birch, rest harrow, wild pansy, knotweed, horsetail, juniper.

❦ GOLDEN ROD–BIRCH–KNOTGRASS COMBINATION ❦

CONDITIONS: Stimulates kidney function, urinary discharge and acts as a mild disinfectant.

DOSE: Pour one pint (16oz) of boiling water over one heaped tablespoon of tea. Allow to steep for 10–20 minutes. Drink a little at a time throughout the day.

CONTENTS: Golden rod (European), birch leaves, knotgrass, horsetail, wild pansy.

COMMENTS: A programme such as the one described in this section causes the loss of many toxic substances through the kidneys. Therefore it is advisable to support, regulate and cleanse the kidneys, best done by sipping small amounts of the golden rod–birch–knotgrass combination tea throughout the day. This formula should not be prepared by boiling but rather by slow steeping. The tea can be taken either cold or warm. If necessary, it can be sweetened with honey, not sugar. It is very important that this tea be taken a little at a time, perhaps a sip every 15–20 minutes. Taken as recommended, this tea will have a generally strengthening and stimulating effect. When combined with the golden rod–silverweed–birch combination and the other three formulae, the body will experience a feeling of renewed strength and well-being.

The person who undergoes a cleansing once or twice a year will experience a general improvement in health and eliminate many substances that might otherwise seriously affect his or her health. The various formulae in this programme not only cleanse and regulate but also help the different organs work in a more harmonious relationship with each other. More frequent cleanses are recommended for individuals suffering from serious constipation problems – perhaps two or three programmes, or until all is regulated, rejuvenated and functioning appropriately. It is very important to take these formulae at the proper times and in the recommended sequences; therefore, pay particular attention to the directions given under each herbal formula heading. This programme, to be effective, should be taken for at least 10–14 days and may be continued for up to three weeks.

USEFUL HERBAL COMBINATIONS

Several herb combinations suggested in the first section are listed below. The principal herbs are given in the heading for each combination. Fresh herb extracts such as these have been used for years in Switzerland, West Germany, the Netherlands, England, France and many other countries throughout the world. In fact, because of their effectiveness, this is the most common way of using herbs in these areas of the world. So when thinking of using herbs, think of fresh herb extracts, where freshness is the difference.

Herbal dosage

The usual dosage for the herbs is 10–20 drops (undiluted or in a little water or juice) three or four times a day. For herbal tablets the dosage is one to three tablets three or four times a day. Some of the combinations listed may have more specific dosages which also may be used if desired. The dosage will need to be tailored to requirements. A child's dosage (under 60 lb) should be half the adult amount.

❦ ARTICHOKE–MILK THISTLE–KNOTWEED COMBINATION ❦

CONDITIONS: Liver and gallbladder cleansing. Stimulates production of bile. Improves digestion of food in the small intestine.

DOSE: 10–15 drops in a little water three times a day (after eating). For some, 5–8 drops may be sufficient.

CONTENTS: Artichoke, milk thistle, knotweed, dandelion root, boldo, barberry, peppermint, aloe, club moss.

ADDITIONAL HERBAL SUPPORT: Aloe–myrrh–cola nut combination (tones the stomach and mildly stimulates bile flow); barberry (gallstones or gravel); dandelion root (improves bile secretion which aids in fat digestion); saffron–aloe–centaury combination (stimulates liver and gallbladder).

❦ BILBERRY–KIDNEY BEAN–ALFALFA COMBINATION ❦

CONDITIONS: A supportive herb combination for cases of diabetes mellitus.
DOSE: Five to ten drops in a little water three times a day (half an hour before eating).
CONTENTS: Bilberry, kidney bean, alfalfa, English walnut, tormentil, cuckoo flower.
ADDITIONAL HERBAL SUPPORT: Dandelion root (improves liver and pancreas function).

❦ COMFREY–WITCH HAZEL–ST JOHN'S WORT COMBINATION ❦

CONDITIONS: Bone, skin and cartilage supplement. Soothes pain in joints. Benefits inflamed mucous membranes in the stomach and intestine. External use will help to regenerate ageing and wrinkled skin.
DOSE: Internally: 5–10 drops in a little water, morning and evening (empty stomach). Externally: apply by rubbing lightly on the affected area, using a liberal amount two to five times a day.
CONTENTS: Comfrey, witch hazel, St John's wort, golden rod (European), sanicle, houseleek, arnica.
ADDITIONAL HERBAL SUPPORT: Comfrey (same use); myrrh (same use).

❦ ECHINACEA COMBINATION ❦

CONDITIONS: Immune system deficiencies, infection, fits and inflammations. Useful for colds and cold-related problems.
DOSE: 15–20 drops in a little water two to five times a day. As a preventative, 10–15 drops twice a day on a regular basis, especially prior to and during the flu and cold season.
CONTENTS: Echinacea herb, echinacea root.
ADDITIONAL HERBAL SUPPORT: Iceland moss–beard moss–plantain combination (colds, coughs, respiratory inflammation).

❦ ENGLISH IVY–THYME–SUNDEW COMBINATION ❦

CONDITIONS: Cough (convulsive), whooping cough and spasmatic cough.
DOSE: Adults: 10–15 drops in a little water several times a day. Children: 4–7 drops in a little water several times a day.
CONTENTS: English ivy, thyme, sundew, coccus cacti, eryngo, ipecac.
ADDITIONAL HERBAL SUPPORT: Pine–sundew–elecampane combination cough syrup (coughs, inflammations of the respiratory tracts); plantain, lance leaf (coughs, congestion).

❦ EPHEDRA–HAWTHORN BERRY COMBINATION ❦

CONDITIONS: Asthma and congestion in the lungs.
DOSE: 10–15 drops in a little water three times a day.
CONTENTS: Ephedra, hawthorn berry, blessed thistle, burnet saxifrage, thyme, gum plant, ipecac.
ADDITIONAL HERBAL SUPPORT: Pine–sundew–elecampane combination cough syrup (coughs, inflammations of the respiratory tract); butterbur (decongestant and antispasmodic for bronchial infections); hemp nettle (expectorant), plantain, lance leaf (congestion and inflammation of mucous membranes of the lungs).

❦ EYEBRIGHT COMBINATION ❦

CONDITIONS: Strengthens and tones the eyes. Eye problems.
DOSE: Internally: 15 drops in a large glass of water and sip throughout the day. Externally: put two or three drops on the closed eyelid and gently massage until fluid is absorbed. Do not allow drops to get directly into the eye, as it will cause a strong stinging sensation.
CONTENTS: Eyebright, chamomile, balm, arnica.
ADDITIONAL HERBAL SUPPORT: Eyebright (strengthens and tones the eyes).

❦ GOLDEN ROD–BIRCH–KNOTGRASS COMBINATION TEA ❦

CONDITIONS: Stimulates kidney function, urinary discharge and acts as a mild disinfectant.

DOSE: Pour one pint (16 oz) of boiling water over one heaped teaspoon of tea. Allow to steep for 10–20 minutes. Drink a little at a time throughout the day.

CONTENTS: Golden rod (European), birch leaves, knotgrass, horsetail, wild pansy.

ADDITIONAL HERBAL SUPPORT: Golden rod–silverweed–birch combination (strengthens kidney and bladder); golden rod, European (strengthens kidney and bladder); stinging nettle (diuretic, gout).

❦ GOLDEN ROD–SILVERWEED–BIRCH COMBINATION ❦

CONDITIONS: Stimulates kidney and bladder function. Useful for kidney and bladder problems and increases urinary discharge.

DOSE: 10–15 drops in a little water three times a day.

CONTENTS: Golden rod (European), silverweed, birch, rest harrow, wild pansy, knotweed, horsetail, juniper.

ADDITIONAL HERBAL SUPPORT: Barberry (kidney gravel); golden rod, European (kidney and bladder function); Golden rod–birch–knotgrass combination tea (kidney and bladder function); horsetail (diuretic); stinging nettle (diuretic, gout); uva-ursi (uric acid, fluid retention, kidney inflammation, kidney stone).

❦ HAWTHORN BERRY COMBINATION ❦

CONDITIONS: Heart tonic. Nervous heart problems, heart stress, palpitations and feelings of anxiety.

DOSE: 15–20 drops in a little water three times a day. It should be noted that hawthorn berry potentiates the action of digitalis, a prescription medicine for the heart. Anyone taking digitalis should keep their doctor informed so that the digitalis medication can be adjusted as necessary.

CONTENTS: Hawthorn berry, oats, valerian, balm, night-blooming cereus, European holly.

ADDITIONAL HERBAL SUPPORT: Hawthorn berry (heart tonic); oats (nerve tonic, lack of sleep); Valerian–passion flower–balm combination (lack of sleep, nervousness).

❦ HAWTHORN BERRY–ARNICA COMBINATION ❦

CONDITIONS: Hardening of the arteries (arteriosclerosis) and signs of senility.

DOSE: 10–15 drops in a little water two or three times a day. It should be noted that hawthorn berry potentiates the action of digitalis, a prescription medicine for the heart. Anyone taking digitalis should keep their doctor informed so that the digitalis medication can be adjusted as necessary.

CONTENTS: Hawthorn berry, arnica, hawthorn blossoms.

ADDITIONAL HERBAL SUPPORT: Herbs and garlic plus vitamin E combination (arteriosclerosis, high blood pressure); bear's garlic (high blood pressure), mistletoe (arteriosclerosis).

❦ ICELAND MOSS–BEARD MOSS–PLANTAIN COMBINATION ❦

CONDITIONS: Colds, sore throat and cold-related illnesses. Helps protect mucous membranes of the respiratory tract.

DOSE: 10–drops in a little water three times a day (half an hour before eating).

CONTENTS: Iceland moss, beard moss, plantain (lance leaf), butterbur, Scotch pine, larch.

ADDITIONAL HERBAL SUPPORT: Echinacea combination (immune support, flu, colds); pine–sundew–elecampane combination cough syrup (coughs, inflammations of the respiratory tract); plantain, lance leaf (cough, congestion).

❦ KNOTGRASS–GOLDEN ROD–BUTTERBUR COMBINATION ❦

CONDITIONS: Arthritic complaints, rheumatism and gout.

DOSE: 10–15 drops in a little water two or three times a day (half an hour before eating).

CONTENTS: Knotgrass, golden rod (European), butterbur,

silverweed, yarrow, birch and leaves, mistletoe, horsetail, meadow saffron, peppermint.

ADDITIONAL HERBAL SUPPORT: Chaparral (inflammation, stiffness); comfrey–witch hazel–St John's wort combination (bone, skin and cartilage support); devil's claw (inflammation); liquorice (arthritis, inflammation); Imperial masterwort (gout, arthritis).

❧ MADDER ROOT COMBINATION ❧

CONDITIONS: Kidney and bladder stones. Urinary gravel.

DOSE: Three to four tablets with a glass of water, immediately after eating. Take for three or four weeks. After a one-week interruption, you may repeat if necessary.

CONTENTS: Madder root.

ADDITIONAL HERBAL SUPPORT: Golden rod–birch–knotgrass combination tea (kidney and bladder function); uva-ursi (uric acid, fluid retention, kidney inflammation, kidney stones).

❧ OATS–GINSENG COMBINATION ❧

CONDITIONS: Strengthens and fortifies the nerves. Useful for stress, restlessness, fatigue, and lack of concentration.

DOSE: 10–20 drops in a little water three times a day (before eating).

CONTENTS: Oat seed, ginseng (*panax*).

ADDITIONAL HERBAL SUPPORT: Siberian ginseng (stress, fatigue), hyssop (fatigue, loss of energy, low blood pressure); oat grass–calcium combination (nervous and mental exhaustion); passion flower (nervous sleeplessness).

❧ POTATO COMBINATION ❧

CONDITIONS: Inflammation of the stomach, gastritis.

DOSE: 10–15 drops in a little water three times a day (before eating).

CONTENTS: Potato herb, potato root.

ADDITIONAL HERBAL SUPPORT: Aloe–myrrh–cola nut combination (tones stomach); centaury (inflammation of stomach).

🦋 SAFFRON–ALOE–CENTAURY COMBINATION 🦋

CONDITIONS: Stimulates liver and gallbladder. Increases secretion of bile in cases of liver dysfunction.

DOSE: Two tablets with a glass of water (after lunch). Gradually increase dosage to four tablets.

CONTENTS: Saffron, aloe, centaury, dandelion root, quackgrass, sarsaparilla, barberry.

ADDITIONAL HERBAL SUPPORT: Senna–buckthorn–aloe combination (stimulates elimination).

🦋 SAW PALMETTO COMBINATION 🦋

CONDITIONS: Prostate problems. Inflammation of the prostate, difficulty in urination due to enlarged prostate.

DOSE: 10–15 drops in a little water three times a day.

CONTENTS: Saw palmetto, golden rod (European), echinacea, aspen, larkspur.

ADDITIONAL HERBAL SUPPORT: Echinacea combination (inflammation); golden rod, European (bladder inflammation); horsetail (prostate inflammation, genito-urinary astringent).

🦋 SENNA–BUCKTHORN–ALOE COMBINATION 🦋

CONDITIONS: Blood cleanser and purifier. Stimulates function of intestines. As a laxative it stimulates elimination without becoming habit forming. This combination also acts as a mild diuretic.

DOSE: Two tablets twice a day (morning and evening). If necessary the dosage may be gradually increased to a maximum of four tablets twice a day (morning and evening).

CONTENTS: Senna leaves, buckthorn bark, aloe, uva-ursi, fennel, chicory, blessed thistle, fumitory, dwarf elder, rest harrow, wild ginger, elecampane.

ADDITIONAL HERBAL SUPPORT: Saffron–aloe–centaury combination (stimulates liver and gall bladder).

TORMENTIL–LOOSE STRIFE–HEMP NETTLE COMBINATION

CONDITIONS: Diarrhoea. Inflammation of mucous membranes of the intestinal tract. Bleeding haemorrhoids.
DOSE: Five to ten drops in a little water three to five times a day.
CONTENTS: Tormentil, loose strife, hemp nettle, knotweed, oats, butterbur.
ADDITIONAL HERBAL SUPPORT: Comfrey–witch hazel–St John's wort combination (soothes mucous membranes in the stomach and intestinal tract).

VALERIAN–PASSION FLOWER–BALM COMBINATION

CONDITIONS: Lack of sleep, sleep disorders, nervousness, stress, mental over-exertion.
DOSE: Lack of sleep: 20–30 drops in three ounces of water sweetened with honey and then drink before going to bed. Nervous stress: 10–15 drops in a little water two or three times a day.
CONTENTS: Balm, oats, passion flower, hops, valerian, hop grains.
ADDITIONAL HERBAL SUPPORT: Oats–ginseng combination (nervousness, stress, fatigue); passion flower (nervous sleeplessness).

HERB AND NUTRITION COMBINATIONS

❦ BEET JUICE CONCENTRATE ❦

CONDITIONS: Anaemia, general weakness. Beet juice fortifies and strengthens the body. It contains many minerals and B vitamins.

DOSE: One tablespoon three times a day (before meals). Beet juice concentrate can be used undiluted or diluted with milk or water.

CONTENTS: Concentrated beet juice. One ounce equals approximately 16 oz of beet juice.

❦ CARROT JUICE CONCENTRATE ❦

CONDITIONS: Vitamin A deficiencies. Benefits intestinal flora and also good for impaired liver functions. An excellent nutritive.

DOSE: One teaspoon three times a day. Carrot juice concentrate can be used undiluted or diluted with milk or water.

CONTENTS: Concentrated carrot juice. One ounce equals approximately 16 oz of carrot juice.

❦ CONCENTRATED LIQUID WHEY ❦

CONDITIONS: Internally: weight control. Helps maintain healthy intestinal flora. Useful for indigestion because it stimulates secretion of gastric acid. Use for sore throat, mouth disinfectant, oral infections and tonsillitis. It increases the effect of rutin. Externally: disinfectant for minor cuts and abrasions. Use for athlete's foot and other skin and nail mould problems.

DOSE: Internally: use undiluted or diluted one to one with water. For a sore throat gargle, mix one part whey to two parts water. Concentrated liquid whey can also be used on salads and in salad dressings as a replacement for vinegar. Externally: for athlete's foot or skin and nail mould mix one part whey to one part water and apply topically.

CONTENTS: Concentrated liquid whey. It contains concentrated amounts of minerals such as magnesium, potassium and calcium.

🦋 HERBS & GARLIC PLUS VITAMIN E COMBINATION 🦋

CONDITIONS: Arteriosclerosis and related complaints such as fatigue, loss of memory, high blood pressure, lack of vitality.
DOSE: One or two capsules three times a day.
CONTENTS: Swiss garlic extract, bear's garlic extract, hawthorn berry extract, passion flower extract, vitamin E.

🦋 OAT GRASS–CALCIUM COMBINATION 🦋

CONDITIONS: Nervous exhaustion. Helps to retain mental and physical activity. Use for overtiredness and general listlessness.
DOSE: One to two tablets three times a day (after eating).
CONTENTS: Calcium, oat grass, glutamic acid, lecithin, natrum phosphoricum, ginseng.
ADDITIONAL HERBAL SUPPORT: Oats–ginseng combination (stress, fatigue); oats (nervousness, insomnia).

🦋 PAPAIN–PAPAYA COMBINATION 🦋

CONDITIONS: Indigestion. Regulator for disturbance of stomach/intestinal secretions. Use for roundworms and pinworms.
DOSE: For digestion, two to three tablets before eating. For worms, four to eight tablets three times a day.
CONTENTS: Papain, papaya leaves, rhubarb root, cysteine, sulphur.

🦋 PINE–SUNDEW–ELECAMPANE COMBINATION COUGH SYRUP 🦋

CONDITIONS: Inflammation of the respiratory tract. Whooping cough, coughs due to colds. Also useful in bronchial asthma.
DOSE: One to two teaspoons every two to three hours.
CONTENTS: Pine juice, sundew, elecampane, English ivy, ipecac, coccus cacti.

❧ PINE EXTRACT COUGH DROPS ❧

CONDITIONS: Mild coughs. Soothing for the mouth and throat. Useful for sore throats.

DOSE: As needed, several times a day. Allow to slowly dissolve in the mouth.

CONTENTS: Raw unrefined sugar, glucose, honey, malt extract, pine bud extract (active ingredient), peppermint oil.

ADDITIONAL HERBAL SUPPORT: Pine–sundew–elecampane combination cough syrup (coughs, inflammation of the respiratory tract).

❧ SEA BUCKTHORN–ORANGE JUICE–MALT LIQUID TONIC ❧

CONDITIONS: Exhaustion, lack of energy. Increases mental and physical capacity. Restores ability to concentrate.

DOSE: One to two teaspoons three times a day. It can be added to fruit juice if desired.

CONTENTS: Sea buckthorn juice (high in vitamin C), orange juice, malt extract, wheat germ extract, date pulp, honey, concentrated grape juice, bee pollen extract, durian (a tropical fruit), yeast extract, rose hip extract.

USEFUL SINGLE HERBS

Many books dealing with the subject of herbs, especially single herbs, may list as many as 30 uses for a particular herb. This only adds to the confusion as to how a particular single herb may be used. With the herbs listed below, consideration is given only to the primary indications of that particular herb, based on the strongest scientific, clinical and folklore use of such herbs.

Both the common name (bold print) and the botanical name (italic in brackets) are listed. A herb may have quite a few common names and many herbs have similar or identical common names, so listing the botanical name will help to determine the proper herb being used.

Fresh herb extracts such as those listed below have been used for years in Switzerland, West Germany, the Netherlands, England, France and many other countries throughout the world. In fact, because of their effectiveness, this is the most common way of using herbs in these areas of the world. So, when thinking of using herbs, think of fresh herb extracts, where freshness is the difference.

Herbal dosage

The usual dosage for the herbs is 10–20 drops (undiluted or in a little water or juice) three or four times a day. For herbal tablets the dosage is one to three tablets three or four times a day. The dosage will need to be tailored to requirements. A child's dosage (under 60 lb) should be half the adult amount.

Alfalfa (*Medicago sativa*)
Antibacterial, arthritis, cholesterol (lowers), oestrogenic effect, nutritive
Angelica (*Angelica archangelica*)
Appetite (improves), colic (baby), kidneys (stimulates), rheumatism
Arnica (*Arnica montana*)
Abrasions, bruises, muscle strain, sprains (external use only for these conditions)
Barberry (*Berberis vulgaris*)
Antibiotic, bile (increases production and flow), candida, gallstones, infection, jaundice, liver disorders
Basil (*Ocimum basilicum*)
Appetite (improves), digestion (aids), urethritis (inflammation of the urethra).

Bear's garlic (*Allium ursinum*)
Antibacterial, antibiotic, antifungal, ateriosclerosis, candida, cholesterol (lowers), colds, fevers, gastritis (inflammation of the stomach mucous lining), heart disease, blood pressure (high), parasites (worms), platelet aggregation, triglycerides (high), yeast infection (urinary and vaginal)

Black cohosh (*Cimicifuga racemosa*)
Blood pressure (high), blood sugar (high, useful for those with high blood sugar or diabetes), cholesterol (high), oestrogen (similar in activity to oestrogen), female tonic, menstrual problems, pregnancy (especially in third trimester), tinnitus (ringing in the ears), uterine disorders, vagina (tones)

Blessed thistle (*Carduus benedictus*)
Anorexia, breast (milk secretion), flatulence (stomach gas, bloating)

Butterbur (*Petasites officinalis*)
Antispasmodic for bronchial infections, decongestant

Calendula (*Calendula officinalis*)
Cramps (menstrual), haemorrhoids, lymph nodes (enlarged), ulcers (duodenal and peptic), varicose veins (combine with witch hazel and apply topically)

Celandine (*Chelidonium majus*)
Warts (external use)

Centaury (*Centaurium umbellatum*)
Anorexia, gastritis (inflammation of the stomach mucous lining), indigestion

Chamomile (*Matricaria chamomilla*)
Anti-inflammatory (reduces inflammation caused by infections, wounds, etc.), flatulence (stomach gas), sclerosis (hardening of tissue and organs), skin disorders, tonic, tumours

Chaparral (*Larrea mexicana*)
Adrenal gland (support), analgesic (pain reliever), cancer, inflammation, rheumatism

Chervil (*Anthriscus cerefolium*)
Blood thinner

Comfrey (*Symphytum officinale*)
Bruises, skin (topical use for healing), sprains, ulcer (peptic), veins (inflamed)

Damiana (*Turnera aphrodisiaca*)
Aphrodisiac (sexual stimulant, especially for males). Works well with saw palmetto

Dandelion root (*Taraxacum officinale*)
Bile (increases production and flow), blood purifier, diabetes,

gallbladder (disorders including gallstones), hepatitis, hypoglycaemia, jaundice, liver disorders, pancreas (tones), skin disorders, spleen (improves function)

Devil's claw (*Harpagophytum procumbens*)
Allergies (mild), arthritis, gout, rheumatism

Echinacea (*Echinacea purpurea*)
see Echinacea Combination on page 164

Eyebright (*Euphrasia officinalis*)
Conjunctivitis (inflammation of the conjunctiva), eye tonic

Garlic (*Allium ursinum*)
see Bear's garlic on page 175

Ginger root (*Zingiber officinalis*)
Circulation (poor), flatulence (stomach gas), motion sickness, nausea, platelet aggregation, stomach (tones)

Ginkgo (*Ginkgo biloba*)
Cerebral vascular insufficiency (poor blood flow to the brain), circulation (poor), memory (loss), phlebitis (vein inflammation), tinnitus (ringing in the ears)

Ginseng (*Panax*)
Adrenal gland (support), fatigue (mental and physical), stress

Ginseng, Siberian (*Eleutherococcus*)
Adrenal gland (support), aphrodisiac, blood sugar (normalises levels), fatigue (mental and physical), mental alertness and efficiency, pituitary (use with liquorice), RNA synthesis, senility (useful with *Ginkgo biloba*), stress, tonic

Golden rod, European (*Solidago virgaurea*)
Bladder (weakness), cystitis (bladder inflammation), kidney (stimulates)

Gotu kola (*Hydrocotyle asiatica*)
Fatigue, memory (mental alertness), stress, tonic

Hawthorn berry (*Crataegus oxyacantha*)
Angina pectoris, arteriosclerosis, cholesterol (regulates), heart (tonic), hypertension, overweight, triglycerides (high), vasodilator (dilates blood vessels)

Hemp nettle (*Galeopsis segetum*)
Asthma, bronchial cough, expectorant

Horsetail (*Equisetum arvense*)
Antibiotic, cystitis (bladder inflammation), oedema (water retention), haemolytic (blood-clotting properties), prostate (enlargement and inflammation)

Hyssop (*Hyssopus officinalis*)
Blood pressure (low), bronchitis

Iceland moss (*Cetraia islandicus*)
Chronic disease states, colds, dyspepsia
Imperial masterwort (*Imperatoria ostruthium*)
Arthritis (mild), gastric and intestinal disorders, gout
Juniper (*Juniperus communis*)
Cystitis (bladder inflammation), kidneys (stimulates), nephritis (kidney inflammation), urinary (antiseptic), yeast infection (urinary and vaginal)
Liquorice (*Glycyrrhiza glabra*)
Addison's disease, adrenal gland (excellent support), arthritis, blood purifier, cirrhosis (prevents), eczema, oestrogen (similar in activity to oestrogen), female tonic, hepatitis, hypoglycaemia, immune system deficiencies, liver disorders, ovulation, pituitary disease (use with Siberian ginseng), respiratory ailments, rheumatism, stomach and intestinal tract (soothes), ulcers (excellent for both peptic and duodenal ulcers), uterus (tonic)
Madder root (*Rubia tinctoria*)
see Madder Root Combination on page 168
Mistletoe (*Viscum album*)
Arteriosclerosis, blood pressure (high)
Myrrh (*Commiphora myrrha*)
Antibacterial, canker sores, gingivitis, leucorrhoea, menstrual difficulties, pharyngitis, yeast infection (vaginal)
Oat seed (*Avena sativa*)
Depression, heart (tonic), insomnia, nervousness
Paracress (*Spilanthes oleracea*)
Athlete's foot (external use), fungus (feet, nail, etc.), gingivitis (swish in mouth), mouth and throat infection (swish in mouth)
Passion flower (*Passiflora incarnata*)
Analgesic (pain reliever), insomnia, sedative, tranquillising
Peppermint (*Mentha piperita*)
Antiviral, colic, flatulence, indigestion
Plantain, lance leaf (*Plantago lanceolata*)
Cough, congestion, earache, lungs (chronic inflammation), respiratory conditions
Red raspberry (*Rubus idaeus*)
Birth (aids parturition), diarrhoea, female tonic, pregnancy, uterus (tones)
Rosemary (*Rosmarinus officinalis*)
Cardiovascular weakness, headaches
Sage (*Salvia officinalis*)
Gingivitis (swish in mouth), mouth and throat

CONCLUSION

Many times on courses or postgraduate lectures, I am asked how I foresee the future of herbal medicine. I usually answer that question by saying: 'Herbal medicine has been around from the beginning of creation and plants have been given to man for healing.'

If we look deep into the resources of the British Museum in London, where Britain's oldest and most precious manuscripts are kept, we can view writings compiled over centuries. It is amazing to read about the wonderful healing methods which were used by our forefathers, whose knowledge we have inherited in these manuscripts. Few people are aware of the existence of these books, let alone have had the opportunity to study them, but the knowledge we can gain from them is considerable. They give us an insight into the medical history of Britain over centuries and describe many natural healing methods which are once more gaining popularity. Often variations of herbal potions have been unjustly seen as placebos. Nowadays, though, we know that herbal potions have been of assistance to many people. The magical workings of extracts and mixtures have been used for centuries to benefit mankind. Much is written about these simple, harmless and generally useful remedies. The primitive physics or the easy and natural method of curing most diseases composed by John Wesley (1703–91) had reached its 21st edition by 1785. All these writings, including today's publications, give us an insight into the tradition of folk medicine. Some traditional British, and especially Scottish, herbs have been used throughout history as home remedies. I not only marvel at their efficacy and suitability for so many purposes, I am also surprised at the quantity. Over the 40 years that I have been in practice, thousands of testimonials from all over the world have reached me. If I am asked whether I believe that there are plants, herbs and roots to cure every illness, my honest answer must be yes. The medicinal properties of plants which grow in the soil are the way to good health. Many people who have gone through the conventional channels with doctors and hospitals, have turned to nature and come to me for advice. They have been able to regain their health, having found an answer to their hopeless suffering with the aid of old, but not forgotten, methods. Looking at some of the writings from the old monasteries or priories, we see that medicinal plants, including beans, savouries, common fennel, sage, mint and a huge variety that is given to us in nature, should be treasured and researched. It is very sad to think that we have spent billions on space investigation, and yet we have not researched all that is growing on earth. If perhaps a fraction of all the money that is spent on medical research had been invested in researching plants, which are freely given naturally, we would have gained a lot more knowledge. The healing properties of digitalis or foxglove were discovered by accident, and haven't they been a blessing to millions of people?

My dear friend, Alfred Vogel, has devoted his life to studying herbs and plants used medicinally, researched them and, with the remedies that he has created, has helped thousands of people all over the world. It is, however, wonderful that, in this present day and age, the younger generation particularly has taken such a tremendous interest in herbal medicine and I am happy that many people are studying methods to heal the body more naturally.

As an external examiner for some of the herbal courses, I have been surprised by the tremendous interest and the quality of work from the younger generation. The course run by Bioforce, which is under medical supervision with two pharmacists involved, has proven to be of interest to pharmacists where guidance for the public is necessary.

Although at the moment there are far fewer plant-based remedies used by medical doctors today than there were over a hundred years ago, it does not mean that they are redundant. There is a dramatic increase in interest by the pharmaceutical industry and they are now taking herbal medicine on board in order to meet the terrific demand from the general public. This is not always for the best, as I still maintain that old studies carried out by specialised people have created responsible products, and the fresher these products are, the better. And that is the reason why I still promote fresh herbal extracts.

Professional reference books are, therefore, necessary, and this book will give some guidance to the complaints that are most common. For as long as this planet has existed, there have been herbs. We have inherited the knowledge from the ancient Egyptians by deciphering old papyrus manuscripts from 2980–2700 BC. Those ancient writings have revealed herbal remedies which have been long forgotten, and prescriptions were made not only for culinary use, but also for medicinal use. The Mesopotamian prescriptions go even further and it is said that in Babylon there was a garden in which 64 species of plants were grown.

China also has an ancient history of pharmacology and modern medicine is indebted to the Chinese for the many plants and medicines which are available.

In India, ancient Hindu philosophy recognised the value of herbal creations, and the principal aim of the ancient Hindu medicine was to prolong life. They also had the idea that fresh plant herbal extracts were the most potent. In their oldest writings, we see how much emphasis was placed on cleansing the body, or detoxifying, which is luckily very much more accepted in today's civilisation.

Hippocrates, the father of medicine, was asked by the Greeks to teach some of the ancient wisdom and he realised only too well how difficult it was to advise medicine for conditions of the time. Claudius Galan (AD 130–201) began as a physician in a school in Alexandria and later was a professor to the Emperor Marcus Aurelius in Rome. He made good use of the writings of Hippocrates and a lot of his expertise became common knowledge.

The Arab religions have a long history and made prescriptions for colonics, going deeply into the philosophies of metaphysics and astronomy connected to the herbs and plants which they produced.

In the Middle Ages, when monks became interested in healing, and even to the present day, we can see the terrific interest that there has been. I visited the excavations of an old monastery on the south side of Edinburgh, and in the apothecary there were still little pots of herbal ointments and herbal medicines to be found, even though this monastery had burned down some time around the eleventh century. A great revolution has taken place since then and it was with the greatest interest that I listened to Alfred Vogel, who had so many of these old writings in his library. It is also very sad that the economy should play such a big role in researching herbs and plants. Because of their popularity, it has been in the interests of certain companies to remove them from circulation in retail outlets such as pharmacies, herbal stores and health food shops, even though these herbal remedies have been proven over the years not to have any side effects.

New discoveries and expeditions are taking place all the time. Herbalism has been here for a long time, even in Britain, and the traditions have stretched back a long way. It is even known that the Druids were skilled in today's remedies like monkshood, primrose, clover, mistletoe, etc.

The father of English botany, William Turner (1520–68), produced writings in the *New Herbal* and gave a lot of information which, luckily, has been saved until today. Another English physician, Nicholas Culpeper (1615–55), produced a lot of controversial writings when he worked with herbs and astrology in a big way. What a joy it was for me to visit Chelsea Psychic Gardens to lecture on the value and properties of the old herbs that grow there. This gives us a picture of the treasures that there are in Britain in the field of herbal medicine. Many books have been written and the *British Herbal Pharmacopoeia*, which is used to train British herbalists, has been accepted all over the world. Herbs which can be used as medicines have also been grown in pots at home on the balcony or in gardens and bear out the promise that was given to man at the beginning of creation, that we would have the fruits to exist and the herbs for healing. Isn't it wonderful to see herbal gardens where people grow their own herbs. Nobody can take away the freedom of choice in what we want to eat or use for ourselves. This is a human right.

Freedom of choice is a wonderful inheritance and, as I have said, this goes back to the beginning of creation, when God calls the Earth to bring forth grass, the herb yielding seed and the fruit tree yielding fruit. There is a treasure of herbs, flowers and plants of which we have gathered so much knowledge over the ages, and they are there for man to use and for the healing of the nations. We can look at herbs and cookery, we can look, too, at garden plants, and we can refer to herbals for medicinal purposes. There are numerous books and writings on herbs such as those written by John Gerard and Nicholas Culpeper published over 300 years ago, giving us hundreds of easy-to-use recipes and interesting and easy-to-grow herbs. The tea mixtures that can be made are numerous and a herbal tea such as the

Dutch Herbal Tea, a recipe from my great-grandmother, is not only helpful but also delightful in taste and smell. In the cosmetic world, there is an enormous range of herbal cosmetics from different sources. I have made a range that is based on the finest of herbs and I have also written a special booklet on it. Going from chamomile, wild pansies, ylang ylang to rosemary and so on, the cosmetic herbal range has, in a short time, made a terrific impact in so many chemists and health food stores as the quality of the product is healthy and safe. Then we look at herbal vinegars, wines, oils, ointments, liniments, poultices, compresses, bubble bath and, in short, all the different extract tinctures, powders, pills, capsules and injections. Too many to write about, and yet, it all comes back to this creation that we are all a part of and which has been tremendously helpful and such a good friend to us.

Today, plant poisons, whether of inorganic, synthetic or plant origin, are under control by the science of toxicology and it is very important that people are aware that self-administered herbal remedies are safe. Unlike synthetic drugs, very few herbal remedies have been totally clinically tested, and it is only because of 40 years' experience that I know what is safe and what is not, mainly because of Alfred Vogel's teachings. I usually say to pregnant women or patients who are on long-term drugs to check with their own doctors or practitioners that it is safe for them to use a herbal remedy. There are some highly toxic plants which I see on the market: although they may be valuable medicinally, they cannot be used without proper medical control. These plants and herbs should be closely supervised and only prescribed with great care. I would like to mention some of the herbs that may cause problems and which should never be collected or prepared for use at home:

Aconitum napellus	(monkshood)
Adonis vernalis	(yellow pheasant's eye)
Arum maculatum	(lords-and-ladies)
Atropa belladonna	(deadly nightshade)
Bryonia alba	(black-berried bryony)
Buxus sempervirens	(box)
Cannabis sativa	(hemp)
Cicuta virosa	(cowbane)
Claviceps purpurea	(ergot fungus)
Clematis recta	(erect clematis)
Colchicum autumnale	(meadow saffron)

Conium maculatum	(hemlock)
Convallaria majalis	(lily of the valley)
Coronilla varia	(crown vetch)
Corydalis cava	(bulbous corydalis)
Daphne mezereum	(mezereon)
Datura stramonium	(thornapple)
Delphinium consolida	
(= *Consolida regalis*)	(forking larkspur)
Digitalis grandiflora	(large yellow foxglove)
Digitalis lanata	(woolly foxglove)
Digitalis purpurea	(foxglove)
Dryopteris filix-mas	(male fern)
Gratiola officinalis	(hedge hyssop)
Hedera helix	(ivy)
Helleborus niger	(Christmas rose)
Hyoscyamus niger	(henbane)
Laburnum anagyroides	(laburnum)
Lactuta virosa	(wild lettuce)
Papaver bracteatum	(Iranian poppy)
Ricinus communis	(castor oil plant)
Robinia pseudoacacia	(false acacia)
Sedum acre	(biting stonecrop)
Solanum dulcamara	(bittersweet)
Taxus baccata	(yew)
Veratrum album	(false helleborine)
Vinca major	(lesser periwinkle)

What a tremendous list of herbs; if we only knew about the thousands of others to be researched.

Pharmacies stock the commercial products, basically packed and pre-packed and under control from the specialist manufacturers. No claims can be made unless the packed or pre-packed medicinal herb has been licensed. However, it is the hope of every herbal practitioner that more money will be spent on research in order to find healing herbs for everyone.

APPENDICES

I: SUMMARIES OF CLINICAL TRIALS OF SOME HERBAL REMEDIES

It is interesting to read some of the reports on well-known herbs that have been criticised for having side effects.

GINKGO BILOBA EXTRACT INCREASES PAIN-FREE WALKING DISTANCE

Patients with peripheral occlusive arterial disease (POAD) in the lower limbs develop intermittent claudication (IC), which limits the distance they can walk without significant pain in the calf. The volunteers recruited in this particular study (63 men and 46 women) had angiographically confirmed POAD (minimum six months) and a pain-free walking distance of less than 150 metres.

The trial was set up as a placebo-controlled, double-blind, multicentre study. Patients were randomised to receive either ginkgo biloba extract (120mg daily) or placebo for 24 weeks.

A walking exercise programme was offered to all patients during the trial period. Treadmill measurements were taken at baseline and after 8, 16 and 24 weeks of treatment. After 8, 16 and 24 weeks of treatment with ginkgo, mean pain-free walking distance increased by 21.2 metres, 31.5 and 45.1 metres respectively, compared with baseline values of 108.5 and 105.2 metres. At all three points the values for ginkgo-treated patients were significantly different from those taking the dummy tablets. No adverse effects were observed for either treatment.

Comment

Intermittent claudication is a common problem in the elderly and may cause loss of mobility, loss of limb and eventually death.

Surgery is possible in some cases to remove the constricted blood vessels in the leg. This study suggests that extracts of ginkgo are useful therapy for IC. Although the improvement noted in this preliminary study may appear small (average 24 metres pain-free walking distances), in percentage terms over the baseline distance of 100 metres, it is clinically significant.

Reference
Peters H., Kieser M., Holscher U. (1998) 'Demonstration of efficacy in Ginkgo Biloba special extract (EGb 761) on intermittent claudication in a placebo-controlled, double-blind, multicentre trial', VASA 27; 106–110.

❧ GARLIC EXTRACTS INHIBIT *HELICOBACTER PYLORI* ❧

Helicobacter pylori is implicated in gastritis, duodenal and gastric ulcers and probably in gastric cancer. Some epidemiological studies have already hinted that a high dietary intake of garlic, and other *Allium*-family vegetables, reduces the risk of gastric cancer. Maceration with oil is a common processing technique used for garlic supplements. The macerate (OMGE) has been shown to inhibit various bacteria (including *H. pylori*) and yeast organisms. The study examined the antibacterial effect of the individual constituents of OMGE against *H. pylori* 'in vitro'.

An OMGE was prepared from fresh garlic using conventional methods and three types of constituents were purified from the mixture. These compounds included ajoenes, vinyldithiins and thiosulphinates. Allicin, which is not a constituent of OMGE, but a thiosulphinate compound, was also studied. All compounds were assessed for their minimum inhibitory concentration (MIC) against three strains of *H. pylori* using standard laboratory methods. The MIC was defined as the concentration of test material that left no microbial survivors.

The result indicated that the ajoenes were active against *H. pylori* with the MIC of 10–25ug/ml. Pure allicin exhibited an MIC of 20–30ug/ml (same range for all thiosulphinates examined), whilst the vinyldithiins had an MIC greater than 100ug/ml and were therefore not regarded as particularly active. All three strains of *H. pylori* were inhibited to a similar extent by the above constituents.

Comment

We can therefore conclude that OMGE contains a number of inhibitory *H. pylori* compounds with 'in vitro' MICs 10–30ug/ml. Not surprisingly, compared to antibiotic preparations these materials appear to be far less potent and therefore not suitable in an acute setting. Amoxycillin, for example, has an MIC of 0.025ug/ml against all three strains from 0.005 to 0.03ug/ml and metronidazole has an MIC of 1.6–3.2ug/ml.

Nevertheless, these results suggest it may be worth while to study OMGE or the individual constituents against *H. pylori* 'in vitro'.

Reference

Ohta R., Yamada H., Kaneko H. (1999) 'In vitro inhibition of the growth of *Helicobacter pylori* by oil macerated garlic constituents', *Antimicrobial Agents and Chemotherapy* 43 (7); 1811–12.

❦ ST JOHN'S WORT HAS FEWER SIDE EFFECTS THAN ORTHODOX ANTIDEPRESSANTS ❦

St John's wort extract (*Hypericum perforatum*) is a herbal remedy that alleviates the symptoms of mild depression and anxiety and, unlike conventional antidepressant medications, is associated with significantly fewer and less severe side effects. The paper by E. Rand *et al* was a systematic review of adverse drug reaction associated with St John's wort from four literature databases plus those sourced from manufacturers, the WHO and the national drug safety monitoring bodies of Germany and the UK. Information on adverse drug reaction originates from case reports, clinical trials, post-marketing surveillance and drug monitoring studies.

Fourteen randomised, placebo-controlled trials were identified where herbal extract was being used to treat depression. The trial period ranged from 4 to 8 and sample sizes from 40 to 120.

In 7 of the 14 trials, no adverse reactions were observed; in 2 trials no information was given, and in the remaining 5 trials 7 patients experienced mild adverse effects. These included unspecified mild stomach complaints, sleep disturbances, nausea, skin rash, itching, drowsiness, reddening of the skin and tiredness. Only in one case of nausea was the adverse effect serious enough to stop treatment. It was also noted that photosensitivity reactions were restricted to acute overdosage with the herb (taken at 30–50 times the recommended dose).

Comment
The balance of evidence is that St John's wort extract has a significantly lower incidence of adverse side effects compared to synthetic antidepressants, although its therapeutic potential is undisputed.

Reference
Ernst E., Rand J.I., Barnes J., Stevinson C. (1998) 'Adverse effects profile of the herbal antidepressant St John's wort (*Hypericum perforatum L.*)', *European Journal of Clinical Pharmacology*; 54; 589–94.

II: ADVICE ON ST JOHN'S WORT (HYPERICUM) PRODUCTS

St John's wort (*Hypericum*) products are unlicensed herbal remedies. Their levels of active ingredients can vary from one preparation to another. They are widely used in the UK, being available from pharmacies, health food shops and herbal practitioners. St John's wort may interfere (interact) with medicines, stopping them from working properly. If a customer is taking medicines, it may be not be safe for him or her to take St John's wort. The advice below is provided to help you understand how this may affect customers.

I AM CURRENTLY TAKING A ST JOHN'S WORT PRODUCT, AND I AM NOT TAKING ANY MEDICINE(S).
🍃 If you buy a medicine from a pharmacy or are prescribed a medicine by your doctor, you must tell your pharmacist or doctor about the St John's wort product.

I AM ALREADY TAKING MEDICINE(S) BUT I WOULD LIKE TO START A ST JOHN'S WORT PRODUCT.
🍃 You must not take a St John's wort product until you have checked with your pharmacist or doctor that it is safe for you to do so.

EPILEPSY OR FITS: I AM ON TABLETS FOR EPILEPSY/FITS AND I AM ALSO TAKING A ST JOHN'S WORT PRODUCT.

TRANSPLANT: I AM ON TABLETS FOLLOWING A TRANSPLANT AND I AM ALSO TAKING A ST JOHN'S WORT PRODUCT.

ASTHMAS OR CHRONIC BRONCHITIS: I AM ON THEOPHYLLINE TABLETS FOR MY CHEST AND I AM ALSO TAKING A ST JOHN'S WORT PRODUCT.

HEART CONDITION: I AM TAKING DIGOXIN FOR A HEART

CONDITION AND I AM ALSO TAKING A ST JOHN'S WORT PRODUCT.

BLOOD CLOTS: I AM TAKING WARFARIN TO THIN MY BLOOD AND I AM ALSO TAKING A ST JOHN'S WORT PRODUCT.

If you have any of the above conditions you will need to stop taking the St John's wort product, as it may stop the medicine from working properly. However, you should see your pharmacist or doctor before stopping the St John's wort product as the dose of your medicine may need to be altered to prevent side effects.

CONTRACEPTIVE PILL: I AM ON THE CONTRACEPTIVE PILL AND I AM ALSO TAKING A ST JOHN'S WORT PRODUCT.

You should stop taking the St John's wort product as it may stop your pill from working. Continue to take your contraceptive pill as normal. There is no urgent need to see your pharmacist or doctor. However, mention it when you next consult your doctor or are dispensed a medicine.

MIGRAINE: I TAKE TREATMENT FOR MIGRAINE AND I AM ALSO TAKING A ST JOHN'S WORT PRODUCT.

DEPRESSION: I AM ON TREATMENT FOR DEPRESSION AND I AM ALSO TAKING A ST JOHN'S WORT PRODUCT.

You should stop taking the St John's wort product as it may stop your medicine from working. There is no urgent need to see your pharmacist or doctor. However, mention it when you next consult your doctor or are dispensed a medicine.

HIV: I AM HIV POSITIVE AND ON TREATMENT AND I AM ALSO TAKING A ST JOHN'S WORT PRODUCT.

You should stop taking the St John's wort product and see your doctor who may suggest you have your HIV viral load checked.

I AM CURRENTLY TAKING BOTH A ST JOHN'S WORT PRODUCT AND A PRESCRIBED MEDICINE NOT MENTIONED ABOVE.

Tell your pharmacist or doctor that you are taking a St John's wort product when you are next dispensed a medicine or consult your doctor.

It is important to always tell your pharmacist or doctor about any herbal remedy or over-the-counter medicine you are taking.

Adrenal dysfunction – abnormal functioning of the adrenal gland.

Ague – a chill; sometimes referring to malarial fever.

Alimentary canal catarrh – inflammation of the mucous membrane of the head, throat, stomach and the lower intestines.

Alterative – blood purifiers; remedies which correct impurities of the blood.

Amenorrhoea – absence or abnormal stoppage of the menses or menstrual periods.

Anaesthetic – a substance or drug that is used to abolish pain.

Anodyne – a pain reliever.

Anthelmintic – something that destroys internal parasites or worms.

Antibiotic – generally refers to an agent that is destructive to bacteria.

Antihaemorrhagic – an agent which stops bleeding.

Antihistamine – an agent which counteracts the capillary dilating action of histamine and causes the capillaries to constrict, thus reducing the amounts of mucous secretions.

Antiperiodic – an agent which controls malarial recurrences.

Antiscorbutic – an effective agent in the treatment and prevention of scurvy.

Antiseptic – a substance or medicinal agent which prevents or destroys micro-organisms responsible for decay or putrefaction.

Antithrombotic – a general term for a naturally occurring substance which neutralises the ability of thrombin, limiting blood coagulation.

Antitussive – relieving or preventing coughs.

Aperient – a mild or gentle purgative.

Aromatic – a substance with a fragrant smell, and which possesses stimulant factors.

Arteriosclerosis – hardening and thickening of the walls of the arterioles.

Arthritis – inflammation of the joints.

Asthmatics – wheezing, coughing and bronchial contractions resulting in dyspnoea (difficult or laboured breathing).

Astringents – agents which cause the tissue to contract. Astringents are vasoconstrictors, inhibiting the bleeding process.

Atonic dyspepsia – lack of strength in the digestive organs.

Atonic leucorrhoea – loss of vaginal tone accompanied by a white viscid discharge from the vaginal area.

Bactericide – an agent which destroys bacteria.

Bronchitis – inflammation of the bronchial tubes.

Canker – a moist open sore, mainly of the lips or gums.

Carbuncle – a mass of dead cells infecting layers of the surface tissue. Usually caused by the bacterium *Staphylococcus aureus*.

Cardiac dropsy – an abnormal accumulation of serous fluid in the heart tissue.

Carminative – relieves stomach or intestinal gases.

Catabolic wastes – waste materials which are produced by the functioning of the body chemistry.

Catarrhal – a word used more frequently by herbalists and natural healers to describe the inflammation and free secretions of the mucous membranes.

Choleretic – an agent which stimulates bile excretion by the liver.

Coagulation – the process of forming a blood clot.

Comminuted – to break or crush into small particles.

Conjunctivitis – inflammation of the thin transparent tissue which surrounds the eyeball. Pink-eye.

Convulsions – a violent, involuntary contraction of the voluntary muscles.

Counter-irritant – a substance or irritation which is intended to relieve some other irritation or pain.

Cradle cap – the build-up of soft tissue on or near the anterior soft-spot.

Croup – an obstruction of the larynx caused by infection and catarrhal discharge.

Cystitis – inflammation of the urinary bladder.

Demulcent – an agent which soothes irritated or inflamed surfaces. A mucilaginous medicine or application.

Dermatitis – inflammation or eruptions of the skin.

Dermatological applicant – a substance applied to the skin surfaces for general beneficial purposes.

Desiccation – to promote drying; loss of moisture due to the drying process.

Desquamation – the shedding of epithelial skin, usually in scales or sheets.

Detergent – an agent which purifies or cleanses.

Detoxifier – a substance which removes or neutralises the properties of a poison.

Diabetes – a disease condition in which the normal body insulin output is in dysfunction.

Diaphoretic – an agent which promotes perspiration or unusually profuse sweating.

Digestant – an agent which assists or stimulates digestion.

Diuretic – an agent which promotes the flow of urine.

Drachms – an older meaning in the apothecaries' system of measurement equivalent to 60 grains (⅛th of an ounce), more commonly called a dram.

Dropsy – the abnormal accumulation of serous fluid in the cellular tissues or in the body cavity.

Duodenal ulcers – cellular tissue breakdown in the first or proximal portions of the small intestine (Latin *duode 'bi*=12 at a time, so called because it is about 12 finger-breadths in length).

Duodenitis – inflammation of the small intestine between the lower end of the stomach (pylorus) and the jejunum.

Dysentery – a condition marked by inflammation of the intestine (usually the colon) with faeces containing blood and mucus.

Dyspepsia – an impairment of the digestive processes.

Dysmenorrhoea – painful menstruation.

Dysuria – painful or difficult urination.

Eczema – an inflammatory skin disease with lesions and watery discharges which usually develops scales or incrustations.

Elliptic – describes the leaf shape, as in the form of an ellipse.

Emetic – an agent which causes or brings on the act of vomiting.

Emmenogogue – an agent that induces menstruation.

Emollient – an agent which softens or soothes the skin or soothes an internal surface.

Emphysema – a morbid condition of the lungs in which they lose their natural elasticity and forced breathing is necessary to fill oxygen requirements.

Endocarditis – inflammation of the inside heart membrane.

Epilepsy – a disease characterised by recurring loss of consciousness, involuntary muscle movements and psychic disturbances.

Excessive menses – an over-abundant bloody discharge during regular menstruation.

Expectorant – an agent that helps the ejection of mucus from the lungs and bronchial tubes.

External abscesses – a localised collection of pus in a cavity formed by the breakdown of tissue on or beneath the skin surface.

Febrifuge – an agent or substance which reduces body fever.

Female climacteric – the critical or turning point in a woman's life in which the psychic and somatic changes occur at the termination of the normal reproductive period.

Fermentative dyspepsia – a condition in which the fermentative process interferes with normal digestion.

Flatulent – distended (filled) with stomach or intestinal gases.

Fomentation – this word is often used to mean a poultice. It specifically refers to the substance applied.

Gastritis – inflammation of the stomach.

Genitals – the male and female organs of reproduction.

Gestation – the period of development from the time the ovum (egg) is fertilised to the time of birth.

Gravel – the coarse concretions (solid mass) of mineral salts formed in the kidney and/or bladder.

Haemorrhage – a large escape of blood from the vessels; bleeding.

Haemorrhoids – varicose blood vessels of the interior anal or rectal cavity. Piles.

Haemostatic – an agent which checks or stops the flow of blood.

Hepatic – pertains to the liver and its proper functions.

Herpes – an inflammatory skin disease with small vesicles formed in clusters. (Cold sore is an example.)

Hydrophobia – old word for the disease rabies.

Hygroscopic – the tendency or ability of a substance to absorb moisture from the air.

Idiopathic headache – headache of unknown origin or cause.

Impetigo – a bacterial inflammatory skin disease.

Indolent ulcers – ulcers which cause only a little pain or discomfort.

Infusion – another term for a tea. Extraction of a medicinal property by using hot, or sometimes cold, water.

Insomnia – the inability to sleep; abnormal wakefulness.

Intercostal neuralgia – pain in the ribs or in the side.

Intermittent fever – a fever that is elevated for a period of time and then temporarily returns to normal; reccurring high and normal temperatures.

Jaundice – a condition of many origins in which there is a deposit of bile pigments in the skin and mucous membranes, resulting in a yellow appearance.

Lactation – the process of giving milk. Suckling.

Lanceolate – refers to the leaf shape being lance-shaped. Four to six times as long as it is broad. Broadest at the base.

Laxative – an agent that acts to promote the evacuation of the bowels.

Leucorrhoea – a whitish sticky discharge from the vagina and uterine cavity.

Lithic material – refers to the calculus or stony build-up in the kidney or urinary bladder.

Mastitis – inflammation of the breast or mammary gland.

Menorrhagia – excessive uterine bleeding; the period of flow between greater than usual or normal.

Metritis – inflammation of the uterus.

Metrorrhagia – uterine bleeding of normal amounts, but occurring at completely irregular intervals.

Mucus (*adj.* mucous) – the free slime secreted by the glands of the mucous membranes.

Myocarditis – inflammation of the muscle tissue of the heart.

Narcotic – an agent that produces a deadening or numbing feeling or condition.

Nephritis – inflammation of the kidney.

Nerve tonic – an agent which tones or strengthens the nerves.

Nervine – an agent which relieves pain (does not include morphine or the narcotics).

Neurotoxic – a poison to the nerve cells or to the nervous system.

Ophthalmia – a severe inflammation of the eye or conjunctiva.

Ovate – a botanical description of a leaf which is egg-shaped.

Palpitation – an unduly rapid action of the heart which is felt by the individual.

Parturient – pertains to the birth process; or sometimes designates a woman in labour.

Parturition – the act of giving birth to a child.

Partus preparatus – an agent which diminishes false labour pains and produces effectual uterine contractions.

Pathogenic – generally refers to an agent which causes sickness or a morbid condition.

Pectoral – pertains to the breast or chest area.

Pelvic neuralgia – pain in the lower part of the trunk or body torso.

Perennial – refers to a plant's life cycle in which it grows year after year.

Pericarditis – inflammation of the membrane which surrounds the heart.

Peristaltic action – the wave-like action of the oesophagus, stomach and intestine which moves alimentary products through the system.

Pleurisy – inflammation of the serous membrane which lines the lungs and thoracic cavity.

Pneumonia – inflammation of the lungs caused by a bacteria in the genus *Pneumococcus*.

Poultice – a soft, moist mass of material applied (usually hot) to the surface of the skin for the purpose of supplying heat and moisture to enhance the healing function of the body.

Pre-parturition – before the actual time of labour and foetal delivery.

Prostatic – pertains to the prostate gland.

Prostatic hypertrophy – a morbid enlargement or overgrowth of the prostate gland.

Prothrombic – pertains to prothrombin, a glycoprotein factor in the blood which is necessary for coagulation (clotting).

Psoriasis – a scaling skin disease.

Pulmonary catarrh – inflammation of the mucous membranes of the lungs and its secretions.

Pulverising – the reduction of any substance to a powder or near-powder form.

Pungent – sharp or biting olfactory sensation. Somewhat acrid.

Purulent – containing pus; or associated with the formation of pus.

Pyorrhoea – virulent inflammation of the membrane which holds the tooth in its socket (periodontal membrane).

Refrigerant – a cooling remedy; an agent relieving fever or thirst.

Relaxant – an agent that lessens tension, especially muscle tension.

Renal antiseptic – an agent which destroyed kidney type bacterial infections.

Renal catarrh – inflammation of the kidney mucous membranes with a free discharge of inflamed mucous material.

Renal cystic – pertains to the kidney and urinary bladder.

Renal mucosa – the mucus-secreting cells which line the kidney ducts, etc.

Renal sedative – an agent which allays or calms the kidneys.

Rheumatic – pertains to the inflammatory condition of the connective tissue structures and of the muscles and joints associated with the tissue.

Rhizomes – these are underground horizontal stems.

Rhus poisoning – poison by touching. Air or smoke contact with the volatile oils of poison oak, poison ivy, etc.

Rubefacient – an agent that reddens the skin (hyperaemia).

Scorbutic disease – a vitamin C-related disease; scurvy.

Scrofula – tuberculosis of the lymphatic glands. Usually a disease of early life.

Scurvy – a vitamin C deficiency disease.

Sedative – a calming agent.

Septicaemia – presence in the blood of bacterial toxins or poisons.

Staphylococcus – a disease bacteria. They are characterised by their clumping formation.

Steep – to soak in a liquid at a temperature under the boiling point.

Stimulant – an agent or remedy that produces stimulation, especially of the muscle fibres through action of the nervous tissue.

Stomachic – an agent or medicine which promotes the functional activities of the stomach.

Stone – a mass of extremely hard material located in the kidney or associated organs.

Strep throat – a sore throat caused by *streptococci* bacteria.

Strobilus – a cone-like reproductive structure bearing spores.

Stye – inflammation of one or more sebaceous glands of the eyelids.

Styptic – an astringent or haemostatic remedy which arrests bleeding by means of its astringent quality.

Suppuration – the formation of pus; the act of becoming converted into pus.

Tetanus – an infectious disease caused by a bacterial toxin which causes sustained contraction of the jaw muscle (lockjaw).
Therapeutic – the art of healing; or to render a cure.
Thyroid dysfunction – an impairment or disturbance in the functioning of the thyroid gland.
Tonic – a medicinal agent or preparation which restores normal tone to the tissue or organ.
Traumatic – pertains to a wound or injury.

Urethritis – An inflammation of the membranous canal which conveys urine from the bladder to the body's exterior.
Uterine subinvolution – failure of the uterus to return to its normal size and condition after normal, functional enlargement.

Vaginal mucosa – the mucous membrane lining of the vagina.
Vaginitis – inflammation of the vagina.
Vasoconstrictor – an agent or substance which causes the blood vessels to become smaller in diameter.
Viscous juice – a juice which has a sticky, thick appearance or property.
Vulnerary – an agent which is active in the healing of wounds.

Weeping eczema – skin inflammation characterised by a watery discharge from the sore or lesion.
Whooping cough – an infectious disease characterised by mucous secretions of the respiratory tract, resulting in a whooping sound.

INDEX

Jan de Vries was born in Holland in 1937 and grew up in occupied territory during difficult war years. Graduating in pharmacy, he turned to alternative medicine where his most influential teacher was the late Alfred Vogel. In 1970 he opened his first clinic in Troon in Scotland and he now also has clinics in Belfast, Dublin, Edinburgh, London and Manchester.

THE

Jan de Vries

HEALTHCARE

SERIES

INNER HARMONY

Jan de Vries

In *Inner Harmony* Jan de Vries explains how we can achieve a
harmonious balance between the three bodies of man – the
physical, the mental and the emotional – to gain optimum
health. Drawing on his vast experience dealing with patients
who have lost their zest for life and joy of living, he is able to
refer to case histories and explain how these problems can be
overcome.

Amongst the problems considered are nervous anxiety, grief,
stress, loneliness, insomnia and resentment – all of them
aggravated by the tensions of living in today's society. The
author refers throughout to dietary management and natural
remedies to help alleviate each health problem. Jan de Vries has
pinpointed many typical complaints of today's living with an
understanding that can only be ascribed to the knowledge that
he has gained in treating thousands of people worldwide.
Written in an easy-to-read style, *Inner Harmony* promotes a very
positive approach to the problems prevalent today.

Available from all good bookshops ISBN 1 84018 062 5
£7.99

THE

Jan de Vries

HEALTHCARE

SERIES

QUESTIONS AND ANSWERS
ON FAMILY HEALTH

Jan de Vries

This is the handbook for every household and is published in direct response to public demand. In this volume Jan de Vries uses all of his vast wealth of experience to answer hundreds of questions which have consistently been asked of him over the years, from varicose veins to the use of vitamin E, headaches to verrucae, from air and water pollution to ME, candida and other present-day problems.

The foreword to this invaluable, easy-to-use reference guide is by Alfred Vogel, author of the million-selling *Nature Doctor* and himself mentor to Jan de Vries.

He is a very balanced, measured man who is totally dedicated to his profession.
Gloria Hunniford

. . . Jan de Vries, 'guru' of alternative medicine, whose methods have helped thousands suffering from conditions of asthma, arthritis, migraines, multiple sclerosis, viruses, cardio-vascular diseases . . .
Marion Pallister, *Evening Standard*

Available from all good bookshops   ISBN 1 85158 587 7
£7.99

THE
Jan de Vries
HEALTHCARE
SERIES

HOW TO LIVE A HEALTHY LIFE

Jan de Vries

How to Live a Healthy Life is an indispensable handbook which outlines the approach to health of one of the world's foremost homeopaths, Jan de Vries.

It gives sensible and easy-to-follow advice on a huge number of subjects, ranging from maintaining a healthy liver and building a strong one to how to follow a well-balanced and nutritious diet and cope with stress.

Dealing with the human body in a holistic way, by considering the three bodies of man – the physical, the mental and the emotional – Jan de Vries advises on osteopathy, homeopathy, naturopathy and phytotherapy, and gives essential advice on how to achieve the healthy lifestyle demanded by the 1990s.

Available from all good bookshops   ISBN 1 85158 754 3
£7.99